How the Brain Makes Decisions

How the Brain Makes Decisions

THOMAS BORAUD, MD, PHD
CNRS-University of Bordeaux

Originally published in French as *Matière à décision* by CRNS Editions, 2015

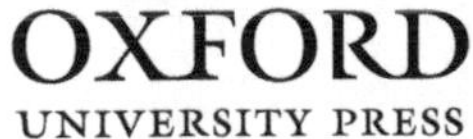

OXFORD
UNIVERSITY PRESS

Great Clarendon Street, Oxford, OX2 6DP,
United Kingdom

Oxford University Press is a department of the University of Oxford. It furthers the University's objective of excellence in research, scholarship, and education by publishing worldwide. Oxford is a registered trade mark of Oxford University Press in the UK and in certain other countries

First Edition published in 2020

Impression: 1

Published in the United States of America by Oxford University Press
198 Madison Avenue, New York, NY 10016, United States of America

British Library Cataloguing in Publication Data

Data available

Library of Congress Control Number: 2020935775

ISBN 978–0–19–882436–7

Printed and bound by
CPI Group (UK) Ltd, Croydon, CR0 4YY

Contents

PART IV. DO COMPUTERS DREAM OF ELECTRIC BANANAS?

PART V. RATIONALITY, FINAL FRONTIER

Introduction to the English Edition

'Fifty Shades of Grey Matter' was, for the sake of witticism, my first choice of title for the English version of this book. It would have been probably better for the press coverage, but it would also have necessitated a twist to the original 'take-home message'. I was considering insisting on the dynamic properties of the brain as a driver of the decision-making process, and how each decision consists of switching from one brain state to the other. Each 'shade' would have corresponded to a brain state and I would have emphasized how aberrant some of those states could be. Unfortunately, even though this argument would have fitted perfectly with the title, I quickly realized that this new orientation was artificial and did not provide a faithful enough rendition of the French version of my essay. So, in lieu of my tentative attempts to be appealing to wide press coverage, I switched to the more straightforward title, 'How the Brain Makes Decisions'.

There are many good books about decision-making that have been published up to now, so why create a new one? The answer to this lies indeed in the title. This book is the first attempt to tackle the neurobiology of decision-making from a 'bottom-up' perspective. I invite the reader on a journey into time, in order to understand from what neural substrate the decision-making structure evolved in vertebrates and how much it impacts on the way we perform decision-making. Therefore, we start from the neural matter and try to understand how decision-making emerged from the physicochemical interactions between its components. This approach is innovative when compared to the traditional view of experimental psychology in which a theoretical principle is enforced into a neural structure using a 'top-down' epistemology.

The French edition was published in 2015 and received honourable press coverage. The distribution and feedback from readers and colleagues allowed me to think that this venture was worthwhile. The text was then re-published in a pocket version. This English edition has allowed me to update my original theory (some predictions I made then have been confirmed since) and correct some errors and approximations (some of which were highlighted by scrupulous readers). I have also updated the historical background (the reader will understand soon that my interest in science is balanced by my interest in

How the Brain Makes Decisions. Thomas Boraud, Oxford University Press (2020). © Oxford University Press.
DOI: 10.1093/oso/9780198824367.001.0001.

history). I rewrote entirely (instead of translating) several chapters, especially the chapters covering pathophysiology, which were too naïve. The revised chapters may still be perceived as naïve perhaps, but I endorse them, and that is not the case anymore for some of my former hypothesis. I have also added a new full chapter about free will. This resulted from discussions, debates and round tables I have participated in since the publication of the original text. These opportunities allowed me to refine my ideas and feel confident to believe that I may have something insightful enough to write about it. Finally, I restructured the book slightly and moved a chapter that was central in the French version into an appendix in the English edition, in order to make the reading easier. In its place I recall the main principle of neural dynamics it relies on. I think this amend is sufficient to understand the main 'take-home message', but I invite any reader who wants to go deeper to have a look at the appendix.

Introduction to the French Edition

Agathe Tyche[1]

With all due respect to devotees of André Malraux,[2] the twenty-first century will be remembered as one of decision-making, and for its new heroes, policy-makers! We are forced to notice that we have totally forgotten that this was not always the case. The concept of decision-making is a Western obsession and one that finally emerged quite late in history. We only have to look to the ancient epics to realize this.[3] Let's take a quick wander through the 'biographies' of Gilgamesh, the heroes of the Mahabharata, or those depicted by Homer:[4] isn't it striking how much they do not seem to act according to their own will, but are guided by external forces?

Even after the emergence of the concept of reason among the Greek philosophers, literature is not immediately permeated by the ancient equivalent of our executive managers. Whether historical figures reported in the annals or fictional characters, they appear to be just as much the play-things of destiny as their pre-Socratic ancestors were. Even if, in his autobiographies, Caesar seems animated by a genuine free will, his famous '*Alea iacta est*', quoted by Suetonius, actually reveals his belief in Fate, just as Demosthenes had engraved his motto on his shield to be placed under the protection of Fortuna. Although imbued with the teachings of philosophers, these political leaders, like most of their contemporaries, were convinced that a higher power was watching over their destiny and dictated their actions. However, this didn't

[1] 'To Good Fortune!' This was the motto of Demosthenes, an Athenian political leader of the fourth century BC. He fought his whole life against the Macedonian expansionism of Philip II, Alexander the Great, and Antipater.

[2] The famous French writer and politician of the twentieth century. He is attributed as saying: 'The twenty-first century will be religious or will not be'. . . I wrote this paragraph in 2013; in light of recent events, he was maybe right, indeed . . .

[3] I voluntary exclude mythological or hagiographical texts that are ontologically disqualified because of their cosmogonic nature.

[4] This list is non-exhaustive. I limited myself to the best known in the Western world. Another interesting example is the one of the Icelandic Sagas. Although, they have been transcript by Christian scholars around the 12th century BC, they refer to ancient myths in which the protagonists are manipulated by the Fate, the central driving force of the Germanic mythology to which even the Gods could not escape.

How the Brain Makes Decisions. Thomas Boraud, Oxford University Press (2020). © Oxford University Press.
DOI: 10.1093/oso/9780198824367.001.0001.

specifically bring them luck: Caesar fell at the hands of the conspirators of the Ides of March, and Demosthenes was forced to take poison. At this time, decision-making capacity was also not the main criteria of popularity for leaders. According to Diodorus of Sicily, for example, the popularity of Gallic kings depended on the harvest. If this was very poor, the king was removed and another was elected.[5]

Christianism did not change this belief. The gallant gesture of the heroes of medieval chronicles simply substituted Faith for Fortuna.[6]

The notion of free will emerges from religious disputes of the Middle Ages, but the heroes of literature have to wait for the reinterpretation of ancient sources through the prism of Christianity by Humanism in order to finally take their destiny in hand. This will result in a new figure immortalized by Shakespeare:[7] the dilemma that strikes those characters condemned to choose between their duty and their emotions.

Following this, decision-making and the motivations that underlie it are increasingly at the heart of the concerns of Western civilization. This is the philosophy of the Enlightenment and its aspiration to universality that will mostly contribute to its spread. It is true that the establishment of democratic regimes presupposes that citizens are rational individuals. Therefore, a value scale between the rational individual (*homo occidentalis*) and the rest of humanity (including women) must be established also. Fortunately, decolonization and feminist movements eventually levelled things and rationality was granted in conjunction with the right to vote for former colonized peoples (who have adopted more or less democratic regimes of their own) and women.

In the twentieth century, choice and commitment, its ideological avatar, replaced fate or faith as principal drives. From initial choice depends the future of the individual in society. For example, French political life still echoes the distant opposition between those who chose collaboration with the occupier and those who chose resistance. Nowadays, the modern hero is the Decision-Maker, the executive manager, the one who makes decisions, whatever they

[5] I have to report something tedious here; I have re-read Diodorus since and have been unable to find this quotation. I am certain I read it somewhere, but I can't remember where and why my memory attributed it to Diodorus. Jean-Louis Brunneau, a French expert in Celtic mythology, cannot either. This given, when we see how much the popularity of modern state leaders depends on the fluctuation of the market on which they have basically no influence, we can ask ourselves whether, behind our supposed rationalism, our deep beliefs are really so far from those of our ancestors?

[6] It is probably one of the factors of the success of the cult of the Virgin that it shares some similarities with Fortuna.

[7] In the French edition I mention Corneille, who wrote his plays about half a century later than the genius of Stratford-Upon-Avon. This was to highlight that in French, 'un dilemme cornélien' became a common phrase.

are. We are imbued with a true mystic of choice. This implies that our decisions should be perfectly rational and reasoned,[8] but nothing is less certain.

My decision to write this book is an excellent illustration. When I took this on, it seemed like a rational idea. It seemed wise to share the knowledge I had gained in the various fields that address the subject and offer my perspective on the neurobiological basis of the selection process.

Then, when the time came to start writing, discouraged by the magnitude of the task, I was less convinced. First of all, my knowledge was not as complete as I had envisaged myself. I had also accumulated a lot of misconceptions. I was hoping it would be easy, I would have plenty of time to devote to the writing, and that I would take pleasure from it. The first two predictions proved wrong. I'm definitely a slow writer and I had to make many sacrifices in order to give myself enough time. In particular, I spent less time with my family and participating in sports activities, while significantly increasing my consumption of tobacco and coffee, which could have an impact on my health. I also wrote fewer research projects and that has significantly reduced funding for my team. In contrast, I've actually enjoyed the process, despite the difficulties and ongoing rewriting. Nevertheless, in making this decision, there have been some negative consequences, and context suggests that the rational decision was to decide not to write this book. However, now that the task is accomplished, I have updated my knowledge and I hope I have corrected at least some of my misconception. It is unclear if the benefit justifies the cost, but that is up to the reader to decide.[9]

Bordeaux, 25 October 2013–Biarritz, 28 September 2014
(for the French edition)

[8] It is even more predominant in France, the motherland of Cartesian rationality!
[9] The feedback received for the French edition, it transpires that the cost/benefit ratio is in fact positive!

PART I

INTRODUCTION

1

Twenty-Five Centuries of Debate

A Short History of Decision-Making

It takes five seconds to decide if you wanna be a problem or if you wanna be a solution.[1]

Introduction

In controlled conditions, it takes only a few tenths of a millisecond to make a decision, but scholars have asked themselves the question of what the underlying process involves since the invention of philosophy, in one of the numerous Greek cities of the eastern coast of Turkey, about 2,700 years ago.

The Beginnings: From Reason to Free Will

The rational discourse, logos (verb) in Greek, preoccupies classical Greek philosophers from Thales to Aristotle and their disciples. It seems that Aristotle was the first to formalize the relationship between decision and logos in *Nicomachean Ethics*. But with the Aristotelian, the concept of logos doesn't dissociate the will driving the reasoning and rationality as we understand it. It is a Latin term (ratio) that will specifically define the faculty of the mind that allows us to fix criteria of truth based on quantification. Between the third century BC and the third century AD, Stoics, who profess that reason must prevail over any other consideration, and Epicureans, defenders of a theory centred on welfare, were opposed in a dialectic that would be summarized in the seventeenth century by Blaise Pascal with its formula: 'the heart has its reasons that reason does not know'. With the advent of Christianism, the debate then

[1] Brother JC Crawford introducing the MC5 before their mythical concert at Detroit in October 1968. In: *Kick out the Jams* by the MC5 (1969).

How the Brain Makes Decisions. Thomas Boraud, Oxford University Press (2020). © Oxford University Press.
DOI: 10.1093/oso/9780198824367.001.0001.

focused around free will after its conceptualization by Augustine of Hippo. Doctors of the church first, then scholastics (Abelard, Buridan, etc.) themselves opposed for centuries using theses, encyclicals, and excommunications as weapons to decide if man is granted with free will and if his actions are predetermined or not. The discussion would be revisited less virulently by humanists (Erasmus, More, Montaigne, etc.) and would ultimately provide ground to the Reformation: between the many griefs that Luther and Calvin carried against the Catholic church, there is the incapacity of its hierarchy to acknowledge that only God saves and free will is an illusion!

Too Much Philosophy Kills Reason

The debate would not come back into the secular domain before the seventeenth century AD, remaining however under the close supervision of the church, which was always ready to excommunicate those who went a thesis too far. In a context where questioning too deeply the central position of man in the creation could bring you to the stake, Descartes buttered up censorship with his famous '*cogito ergo sum*'.[2] It defines man through self-awareness and creates the dichotomy between man, the only true thinking being, and the rest of the animal world. It influenced the Western world's philosophy to such an extent that Cartesian dualism is still prevalent today. Proponents of the theory of mind concede self-awareness to all animal species able to recognize themselves in a mirror (which includes apes,[3] orcas, elephants, and magpies),[4] but many are those who violently oppose and deny the existence of non-conscious decisions. Amazingly, fundamentalists of Cartesian dualism are recruited from within scientists, Lacanian psychoanalysts or religious extremists of any obedience. From this point, philosophers slowly turned away from the debate of free will and reason itself to focus rather on the ethics of action, like Spinoza, or the application fields of rationality (Kant).

Blaise Pascal, who was both a philosopher and a mathematician, and who lived at the same time as Descartes, not only summarized the old debate between Epicureanism and Stoicism but also drove the issue of reason out of the muddy field of speculation to enter the rigorous world of mathematical formalism. His famous wager on the existence of God introduced the use of

[2] Translation: 'I think therefore I am'.
[3] This category includes bonobos, chimpanzees, gorillas, orangutans, and gibbons.
[4] In humans, self-awareness appears between 6 and 12 months (Wallon, 1934).

probabilities to make a decision in a context of uncertainty. For Pascal, it could be solved as follows: If I bet that God exists, at best (if He exists), I gain eternal life; at worst (if He doesn't exist), I lose the pleasures of earthly life, which Pascal considered negligible. If I choose not to believe in God, my maximum loss is eternal damnation. So, for Pascal, to believe in God minimizes losses, therefore it is the only reasonable option. This wager[5] is the origin of the mathematical formulation of the problem of decision-making, regardless of its theological implications. Pascal speaks for himself only concerning the values he attributes to eternal life as compared to the pleasures of earthly life! In the mid-twentieth century BC, von Neumann formalized this approach with the minimax theorem to determine, in a two-dimensional matrix of losses and gains, what is the least costly solution for decision-making in uncertain conditions. It is rare, however, for the issue to be as dramatic as when one plays his soul against God!

The Day Economics Replaced Philosophy

The formalistic approach inspired the Swiss mathematicians, who, pragmatically, were more concerned with economic risk than the salvation of their souls. The most famous of these was the Bernoulli[6] family including Daniel,[7] a descendant of the second generation, who introduced the concept of utility,[8] a mathematical function of the value attributed to property by a subject that varies depending on the risk associated with obtaining it (see Figure 1.1). It provided a tool to quantify the notion of subjectivity of needs at the core of Market theory. Economics emerged from the Enlightenment era with the systematization of these principles by Adam Smith.[9] The Scotsman categorized the key parameters that influence the subjective feeling of needs and thus constrain the behaviour of choice and aggregation of individual behaviour

[5] The original formulation is as follows: You have two things to lose, the true and the good; and two things at stake, your reason and your will, your knowledge and your happiness; and your nature has two things to shun, error and misery. Your reason is no more shocked in choosing one rather than the other, since you must of necessity choose. This is one point settled. But your happiness? Let us weigh the gain and the loss in wagering that God exists. Let us estimate these two possibilities. If you gain, you gain all; if you lose, you lose nothing. Wager, then, without hesitation that He exists (Pascal, translated from the French edition).

[6] A family of Swiss scholars and artists who produced several mathematicians over two generations between the seventeenth and early eighteenth century AD, whose work has had numerous applications in physics and economics.

[7] Daniel Bernoulli (1700–1782) was also an innovator in the field of fluid mechanics.

[8] Readers could refer to the glossary at the end of this book.

[9] Adam Smith (1723–1790), is considered as the father of modern economics with his book entitled *An Inquiry into the Nature and Causes of the Wealth of Nations* volume I (1776). He died before writing volume II.

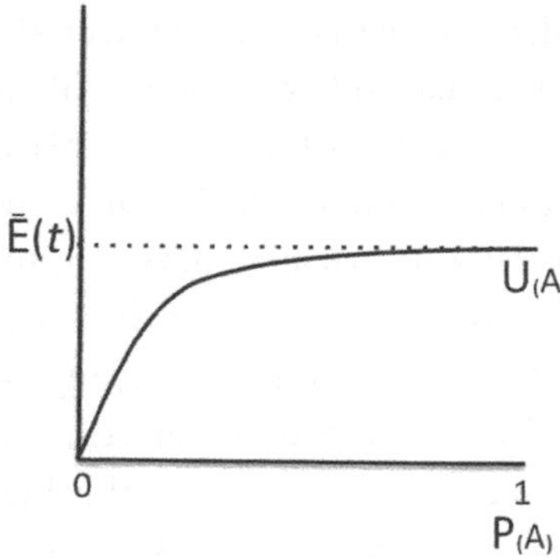

Fig. 1.1 Utility function. Given a set of lotteries with a fixed expected value ($\bar{E}_{(A)}$ = Probability × Value) but different probabilities (therefore the values are also different in inversed ratio). Utility $U_{(A)}$ as defined by Bernoulli is asymptotical to $\bar{E}_{(A)}$ when $P_{(A)}$ is high but is far from it when $P_{(A)}$ is low. This function matches well with the behaviour of subjects that prefer options with lower expected value but are less risky. We call this behaviour, frequently observed, risk aversion.

in economic activity. From this time, the question of the formalization of the principles of decision-making never left this field and is still at the heart of the concerns of several schools of economists.

Amongst others, let's mention quickly the works of Samuelson[10] and Houthakker,[11] who defined the notion of revealed preference that infers the tastes of subjects from their choices rather than from what they say. Here is a classic example: If we ask a subject to choose between an apple and a banana and he chooses the banana, then it infers that he prefers bananas to apples. This approach is particularly valuable because the post-hoc justification of a choice by a subject is notoriously unreliable;[12] overall it also enables us to study the preferences of subjects who are unable to justify their choices verbally (such as infants and animals). The next step was taken by von Neumann and Morgenstern[13] who brought both the work on utility and that on revealed preferences together, and developed an axiomatic approach to decision-making uncertainty. According to their theory of expected utility, when faced with a choice (A, B, or C) of different utility $U_{(A)}$, $U_{(B)}$, or $U_{(C)}$, a rational individual

[10] Samuelson (1938).

[11] Houthakker (1950).

[12] Pareto (1848–1923) even wrote 'economy will have a great interest to depend as least as possible of psychology'. He referred to the Mentalist school based upon introspection.

[13] von Neumann and Morgenstern (1944).

must meet four conditions: i) completeness (given two options A or B, a subject must prefer A to B, B to A, or have no preference); ii) transitivity (if he prefers A to B and B to C then he must prefer A to C); iii) independence (if he prefers A to B, then regardless of the lottery C and the probability p between 0 and 1, this subject should prefer p.A + (1-p).C to p.B + (1-p).C]; and finally iv) continuity (if he prefers A to B and B to C, then there must be a probability p between 0 and 1 for which B = p.A + (1-p).C.

Rats, Pigeons, and Armed Bandits

Under the influence of Positivism in the late nineteenth century, economists were joined by psychologists who arrived at the same conclusion on the need to study the process of decision-making by emptying it of any mentalist consideration. Thorndike[14] raised the principle of reinforcement learning, which states that if a behaviour is followed by a reward repeatedly, then they will eventually be associated. This opened the way to behaviourism,[15] which dominated the field of experimental psychology throughout the twentieth century and is still particularly influential. Skinner[16] radicalized the concept of association between an action and reinforcement by defining operant conditioning. To illustrate this concept, the easiest way is to borrow an example from Skinner himself: Take a lab rat, put it in a box (now bearing the name of Skinner's box) that includes levers and a food pellet dispenser. If, when the animal presses a lever, a food pellet is issued, he will learn to associate his action on the lever with the reward, meaning that for the majority of the time he will spend in the box, he will run back and forth between the lever and the pellet dispenser. The rat's behaviour will be conditioned by the reinforcement. This method of investigation would be developed, advanced, and adapted to study the learning process in almost all species, from earthworm to human.

An interesting, because it is a more ecological, alternative is to associate the action and the reinforcement according to a certain probability. In experimental psychology, we talk about the contingency rule (the term is borrowed from statistics). It is close to the principle of the slot machine, which is to operate a lever (or push a button for the newer versions) for a monetary reward.[17]

[14] American Psychologist (1874–1949), precursor of behaviourism.

[15] This neologism was invented by Watson (1878–1858) in order to label the branch of psychology that studies how the environment and the history of a subject influences their behaviour.

[16] Burrhus Frederic Skinner (1904–1990) was the most radical behaviourist.

[17] In fact, slot machines are a bit more complex: the probability of winning the jackpot depends on the number of winning combinations divided by the total number of possible combinations (it is therefore

The stronger the contingency, i.e. the more likely the action is to lead to a reward, the faster the learning will be. This experimental paradigm responds to the gentle name of the One-Armed Bandit task. This type of protocol enabled Rescorla and Wagner to formalize the learning law of a subject from the difference between the expected result and the actual result.[18] This postulate with high heuristic value has been very influential in experimental psychology over the last 40 years. It is also very similar to the concept of expected utility that we encountered in economics, and marks the beginning of a convergence between the two disciplines.

A decisive step in the study of decision-making would be reached by a student of Skinner, Richard Herrnstein (1930–1994) who worked with pigeons. He developed a variant of the One-Armed Bandit task that became the benchmark of the paradigm to study decision-making.

It was called the Two-Armed Bandit task by analogy (see Figure 1.2A).[19] In it, the subject is confronted with two options. Each option has a fixed gain (e.g., a seed for birds)[20] but different probability of reward ignored by the subject. The subject is entitled to a number of successive attempts (between tens to hundreds depending on the experimental protocols) during which he must choose one of two options. To an outside observer, it is possible to infer the expected utility ($\bar{E}$) for each option by computing the ratio between the number of times the option was awarded and the number of trials performed. The work of Herrnstein helped to formalize a concept still widely discussed in the literature: the balance between exploitation and exploration. A subject exploits their environment when they show a marked or exclusive preference for the most attractive option. A subject explores when they show no preference for one of two options. Herrnstein found that pigeons chose proportionately to the contingency rules of the two options he proposed (see Figure 1.2B). It never follows the most rational solution which would have been to exploit, i.e. select only the best-rewarded option. Surprisingly, this lack of rationality that one can expect from pigeons devoid of a proper cortex (but see Chapter 7), is found

fixed ... in theory). The magnitude of the gain is set by the compensation rate. The latter, which is a minimum imposed by law (in France it is 85 per cent) defines the amount of money that must be redistributed to the customers of the casino over a given time. Therefore, the amount won for a jackpot depends on the history of the machine.

[18] Rescorla and Wagner (1972).

[19] The test was used in a wide variety of species, including the pigeon (favoured by Herrnstein), crows, coyotes (!), various species of rodents, and primates including apes and humans.

[20] The nature of the reward varies depending on subjects. In animals, it is usually a food reward (solid or liquid); in humans it is usually a monetary reward (although food and sex have also been proposed by playful experimenters).

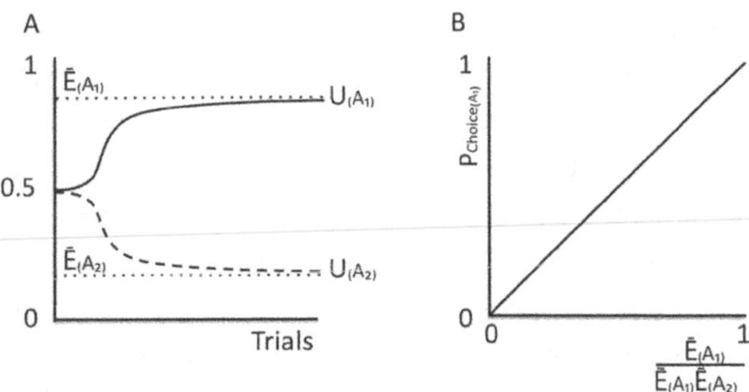

Fig. 1.2 Two-armed bandit task. (A) The subject has the choice between two lotteries A1 and A2 of different but unknown expected value (here $\bar{E}_{(A1)}>\bar{E}_{(A2)}$). The utility (U) of the two lotteries is similar at the beginning, but after each trial, the outcome of each choice allows subjects to revaluate $U_{(A1)}$ and $U_{(A2)}$ that became asymptotic to $\bar{E}_{(A1)}$ and $\bar{E}_{(A2)}$ respectively. Once expected value has been approximated, a rational subject is supposed to choose exclusively the best option (A1 here). The problem is that this is seldom the case. **(B)** Herrstein matching law is a blatant demonstration. When this task is proposed to pigeons, their probability to choose the best option $P_{choix(A1)}$ is proportional to the expected value of A1 divided by the sum of all the possible expected values. At variance with what we can expect, humans perform as pigeons in this task.

in all species that have been tested with this type of protocol, including apes and humans.[21]

Economics Trapped in Contradictions

This finding is just one example among many of the limitations of rationality. Economists have come to the same conclusion as the behaviourists evidencing a number of paradoxes by following a different thread. One of the best known is the paradox of Maurice Allais, a French Nobel Prize winner in economics,[22] highlighted at a conference which brought together the crème de la crème of the discipline in 1952. He proposed to his colleagues that they choose

[21] See (non-exhaustively): Herrnstein (1974); Graft et al. (1977); Bradshaw et al. (1979); Matthews and Temple (1979); Dougan et al. (1985); Herrnstein et al. (1989); Lau and Glimcher (2005); Morris et al. (2006); Pasquereau et al. (2007); Lau and Glimcher (2008); Gilbert-Norton et al. (2009); and Palminteri et al. (2009).

[22] In fact, of the exact name is Swedish National Bank's Prize in Economic Sciences in Memory of Alfred Nobel. The prize was established in the late sixties and is highly controversial.

between lottery A, consisting of a 100 per cent chance to win 10,000 FF,[23] and lottery B, consisting of a 90 per cent chance to win 15,000 FF.[24] Although the Expected Value of lottery B is greater ($\bar{E}_{(A)} = 1 \times 10{,}000 = 10{,}000$ FF; $\bar{E}_{(B)} = 0.9 \times 15{,}000 = 13{,}500$ FF, a computation that any undergraduate in economics knows how to do!), most of his fellows chose lottery A. This behaviour is known as risk aversion (see Figure 1.1). In other words, although $\bar{E}_{(A)}$ is less than $\bar{E}_{(B)}$, the utility $U_{(A)}$ is greater than $U_{(B)}$. The paradox comes from the second proposal made by our playful economist. He offered them two new lotteries; lottery C, consisting of a ten per cent chance of winning 10,000 FF, and lottery D, consisting of a nine per cent chance of winning 15,000 FF. Here the choice made by the majority of his colleagues was for lottery D, of which the Expected Value ($\bar{E}_{(D)} = 1{,}350$ FF) is actually higher than that of lottery C ($\bar{E}_{(c)} = 1{,}000$ FF). But, C can be decomposed into p.A + (1-p).Z and D into p.B + (1-p).Z with p = 0.1 and Z being a lottery of Gain = 0. Our prestigious assembly of economists therefore violated the principle of independence, which is one of the four founding axioms of their discipline. The reasons for this paradox are still being debated. Leonard J. Savage, a famous American statistician who was present, claimed that it was because of the wine that had been served at lunch (the conference was happening in France, so much for the cliché!). However, when these scenarios are reproduced with a panel of sober subjects, the results are consistent. This was the first demonstration that constraints limit the ability to reason rationally, even among experts.

Rationality, Final Frontier

Thus, behaviourists and economists reached almost simultaneously the limits of rationality in the second half of the twentieth century. For the former, it could be perceived simply as an interesting phenomenon per se; but for the latter, it generates a real existential crisis: How do we identify general principles that govern the world economy, if the decisions that are the source of their fluctuations are not based on rational foundations? Would economics be the victim of its own contradictions? As is so often the case, salvation has come from inter-disciplinary approaches. Inspired by information theory,[25] Simon[26]

[23] For French Francs; the FF was devaluated in 1958 so 10,000FF approximates 12 £ today (without adjustment to the cost of life).

[24] The attentive reader will notice that we are in a scenario close to a One-Armed Bandit task except that in experimental economics lottery probabilities are provided explicitly.

[25] Shannon (1948).

[26] Simon (1947). Herbert Simon (1916–2001), Nobel Prize in economics in 1978.

defined the principle of bounded rationality. For him, the main cause of the limitation of human rationality is that our brain is unable to handle the mass of information available. This approach opens the way to a mathematical formalism that aims to maximize performance based on the quantification of the amount of information available.

Rationality in Prospect

However, other causes have been identified. Daniel Kahneman and Amos Tversky, two Israeli experimental psychologists, scrutinized the cognitive biases that are the foundations of the paradoxes observed in experimental economics. One of their most famous experiments has shown the extent to which how a problem is formulated then influences the choices made by its subjects. Their seminal experiment consisted of offering two groups of students the following dilemma: Which policy to choose within the framework of an epidemic that erupted in their country. To one group they asked them to choose between saving 200 people out of 600 with certainty (policy A), or, with a probability of one-out-of-three, to save 600 people (policy B). The question was then phrased differently to the other group: Choose between leaving 400 people to die without fail (policy A'), or, with a probability of two-out-of-three, choose to see 600 people die (policy B'). Interestingly, the Expected Utilities of all these solutions are the same (on average 200 people will be saved), so there is no single 'better' policy. In addition, policies A and A' differ only in their formulation, and this is the same for policy B with respect to policy B'. The subjects of the first group favoured A due to risk aversion (they are certain to save 200 people) while the second group favoured B', which suggests the possibility of saving 600. They called this cognitive bias 'framing'. From these observations, Kahneman and Tversky proposed Prospect Theory, which formalizes how subjects rate loss and gain with asymmetric prospects.[27] This theory postulates that individuals define their preferences with respect to a reference point (frame) from which the subject will evaluate the gains (which are above) and losses (which are below). The value (V) binding the subject's preference to results does not follow the same laws for the gains and the losses. It is concave for the former and convex for the latter, and the slope of the loss is greater than that of the gains (see Figure 1.3A). This asymmetric sigmoid function accounts for the sensitivity to losses. This function is then weighted by a factor 'w' to set the

[27] Kahneman and Tversky (1979).

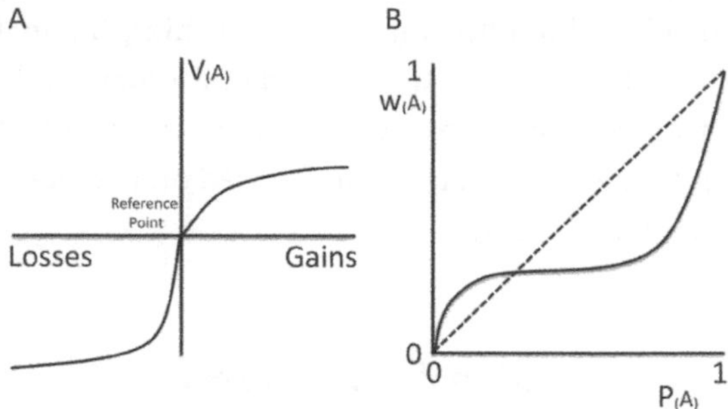

Fig. 1.3 Prospect theory. (**A**) Value granted to options depends on a framing point. The slope of the loss curve is steeper than that of the gains. (**B**) The pondering factor $w_{(A)}$ used to compute utility ($U_{(A)} = w_{(A)} \times V_{(A)}$) is a non-monotonic function of $P_{(A)}$. Individuals overvalue small probabilities and undervalue large ones. Adapted from Kahneman and Tversky (1979).

utility ($U = w.V$) from which subjects choose. This weighting factor reflects the tendency to overestimate low probabilities and underestimate high probabilities (see Figure 1.3B).

Kahneman and Tversky thus explain why the choices of their subjects are in contradiction with the axiomatic approach of Von Neumann and Morgenstern. They also solve at the same time a number of paradoxes, including the Allais paradox. This theory is behind the behavioural economics that was consecrated by a Nobel Prize in Economics awarded to Kahneman[28] in 2002. Since then, many studies have followed and new biases have been identified and formalized. They involve memory, reasoning, and emotions, of course, but also the personality of the subjects. For example, a series of recent studies, initiated by Tali Sharot,[29] shows the influence of optimism on our daily decisions. One of the most striking examples, which she used to quote in her lectures, is a study on marriage, whose participants consisted of a group of London lawyers who specialized in Family law. The question was posed to those who were to be married, in the month preceding the ceremony, to estimate the likelihood of them divorcing within the ten years that followed. Their answers revealed a pleasing corporatism of spirit, since they all replied without exception, 'zero per cent'. Knowing that, in London, the divorce rate after ten years of marriage

[28] Tversky died in 1996, he thus cannot benefit from the Nobel Prize, the rules of which stipulate that it cannot be awarded posthumously.

[29] Sharot (2011).

is between 30 to 40 per cent, as in all European capitals, this example demonstrates how optimism can skew judgement.

And the Brain in All of This?

This review is far from comprehensive, but its goal was to bring the reader to the conclusion that more than 25 centuries after the emergence of the concept of reason, psychologists and economists agree that the concept of rationality is relative. To grossly summarize: When a subject decides, he doesn't usually optimize choice. For behaviourists, explanation is to be found in exploratory behaviour. Evolutionary pressure has selected behaviours that anticipate possible changes in environmental conditions. The subject (animal or human) exchanges some immediate efficacy against information which may serve him later. For economists, the answer is more complex. It is a combination of the inability to understand all of the options surrounding a problem (bounded rationality) associated with biases that cloud judgement.

But what about the organ of decision-making? What can study of the brain tell us? Can we unravel the mechanisms that underlie these theoretical concepts (exploration, exploitation, bounded rationality, and cognitive biases)? This is the goal of this text, starting from the fundamental question: What are the basic properties that a neural network of decision-making needs to possess? We will use a bottom-up approach of the neural substrate of the decision-making process. Combining data drawn from phylogeny and physiology, we will draw together a general framework of the neurobiology of decision-making in vertebrates and explain how it evolved from the lamprey to the different taxa of vertebrates, including apes. We will then address the consequences: how it impacts our capacity for reasoning, and examine some aspects of the pathophysiology of high brain functions. In conclusion, we will open up discussion to more philosophical concepts.

2

A Ghost in the Machine

The Neurobiology of Decision-Making

In this case you will declare: he is one who has a wound at his temple, penetrating the bone, (. . .) who has blood coming out of his nostrils, who had a rigidity of his neck, one who is voiceless. This one, is one I cannot heal.[1]

The Eye of the Clinician

This passage from the Edwin Smith papyrus is often quoted as the first description of traumatic aphasia attesting that, as far back as the Bronze Age, Egyptian physicians would have noticed the link between the jelly pudding contained in our skull and cognitive abilities. However, even considering the archaism of the language, it is not certain that we can assimilate 'one-who-is-voiceless' with aphasia. But, in other passages of the same papyrus, a lesion of the viscera-of-the-head (the brain!), following a traumatic injury, is associated with motor impairment. It is therefore clear that the Egyptians had identified the role of the brain at least as a prime mover.

The Greek world had to wait until the dissections of Herophilus of Alexandria (fourth to third centuries BC). Until then, following Hippocrates, they tended to locate the logos in the heart under the control of the humours. Both theories long remained in competition. During the 20 centuries that followed, knowledge advanced slowly thanks to the propensity of Homo sapiens to smash the skull of his fellow contemporaries by all possible means. This occurrence graciously provided practitioners with numerous clinical cases of brain damage to observe. More contributions were made through dissections usually done in secret by the church,

[1] Edwin Smith papyrus (seventeenth century BC), personal translation. I know, the grammar is awkward, but my teacher emphasized the necessity of maintaining the archaism in the translation in order not to betray the ancient Egyptian way of thinking.

How the Brain Makes Decisions. Thomas Boraud, Oxford University Press (2020). © Oxford University Press.
DOI: 10.1093/oso/9780198824367.001.0001.

always prone to incinerate body-snatchers. In the nineteenth century, Positivism reached medicine and practitioners began to try to connect more or less focal lesions with deficits measured more precisely using standardized tests. They focused naturally on the motor and sensory functions that are easier to objectify. Phineas Gage is a famous exception. This unfortunate worker of the huge railway construction project, joining together the east and west coasts of the United States, was seriously wounded in 1948 after mishandling explosives. A metal rod went through his left frontal lobe. He miraculously survived this tragic accident and seemed not to have suffered motor sequelae, but his personality seems to have been significantly altered. He became unstable, rude and capricious whereas he had been considered as quite puritanical before the accident. The case of Phineas Gage, reported by Harlow (1819–1907), is considered to be the first case report of a personality change following a brain injury. The association of this change with frontal lobe lesions was completed in 1994 by Antonio Damasio and Antoine Bechara[2] after having exhumed the skull of the unfortunate and proposed a reconstruction of the extent of the lesion by modern imaging methods.

It was also in the middle of the nineteenth century that practitioners came to realize that rather than waiting for fate to provide subjects with brain damage, lesions could perhaps be induced in animals. This was the birth of experimental neuroscience.

The Miracle of Electricity

The physiological approach made a fundamental advance after the discovery of the electrical properties of neurons. In the mid-nineteenth century, Emil du Bois-Raymond (1818–1896), a German scholar, was the first to identify the spikes: electrical events, invariant in shape and amplitude,[3] which propagate along the axons of neurons. Louis Lapicque (1866–1952), a French physician and physiologist, defined the conditions under which this signal propagates from one neuron to another. He was also the first to propose a mathematical model of neurons called 'integrate and fire' that is still used today. Integrating electrical stimulation and lesion, Sir David Ferrier (1843–1928) established the first functional brain mapping (mainly motor areas) in dogs and primates. This was complemented by the work of the first electrophysiologists who sought to correlate brain activity with behavioural observations (sensory stimuli,

[2] Bechara et al. (1994); Bechara et al. (1996); Bechara et al. (2000).

[3] In fact, when neurons fire in bursts, the amplitude of spikes tends to decrease.

movements, etc.). Their approach was macroscopic at first, with the development of the electroencephalogram recording the changes of electric potentials on the surface of the skull. Microelectrodes were then used to obtain a better resolution down to the scale of the neuron. Applied at the sensory and motor areas of the cortex, single neuron electrophysiology identified the main principles of coding of information by these structures in the second decade of the twentieth century. This allowed us to infer that most of the information is contained in the neuron firing rate, i.e. the number of spikes per unit of time.

And Neurons Predicted Choice!

Until the late 1980s, ignoring the work of experimental economists and behaviourists, electrophysiologists restricted themselves to the study of sensory and motor function, believing it to be impossible for them to access cognitive processes. In 1989, William Newsome and Anthony Movshon broke the dogma while studying the role of neurons in the medio-temporal area of the cortex (an associative visual area) in the visual discrimination of macaques. The task consisted of watching dots that move randomly on a screen (see Figure 2.1).[4]

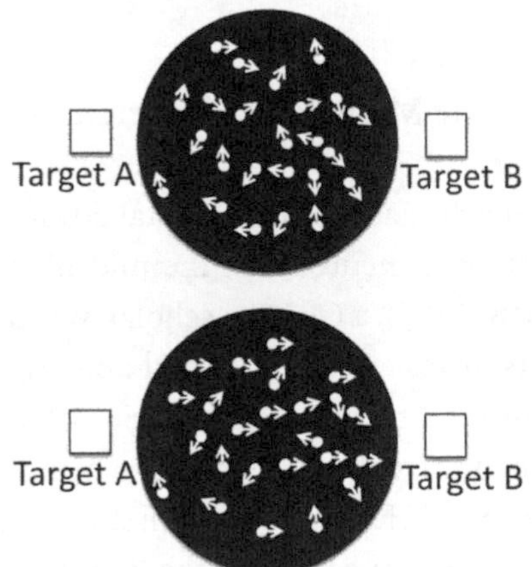

Fig. 2.1 The random dot experiment. The subject is seated in front of a screen on which dots move. Targets are located on each side of the screen. The subject must fixate his gaze if the dots are moving completely randomly. If he detects an apparent movement (as in (B)), he must operate a saccade toward the corresponding target. In experimental conditions (with many more dots), animals can detect a movement from 3 per cent of coherence.

[4] Newsome et al. (1989).

Within this population, a small fraction moves in the same direction. To investigate the capacity of discrimination, experimenters vary the level of consistency, i.e. the proportion of dots that move in the same direction. To check whether the animal was able to distinguish an apparent motion, they encouraged it to indicate by a saccade the direction in which the dots animated with a coherent movement were heading. This study produced two surprising results. The first was that the animals were able to discriminate an apparent movement below three per cent consistency, and the second, most pertinent regarding our own line of interest, was that the firing activity of the neurons of the medio-temporal cortex area anticipated the choice made by the animal. Newsome and Movshon therefore stepped into the history of the neurophysiology of decision-making as the pioneers who first managed to correlate decision-making with electrophysiological activity in neurons. This correlation, which they called psychometric–neurometric pairing, became the backbone of all subsequent studies of the neurobiology of decision-making. The discovery was fortuitous: for them, the decision-making of the animal was a way to check the direction of apparent motion discriminated by the animal. From then on, the electrophysiological community realized that the study of the neurobiological correlates of decision-making was now within reach.

When the Brain Lights Up, Phrenology Is Not Far

The next step was the development of functional MRI, in order to visualize in 3D using a spatial resolution to the order of a cubic millimetre, changes in cerebral blood flow. The signal captured is known as BOLD, which stands for 'blood-oxygen-level dependent'. It is correlated to variations of glucose and oxygen consumption in brain tissue that indirectly reflect the activity of neural populations with a delay of about a second. Although this method provides indirect information and poor temporal resolution, the disadvantages are outweighed by its non-invasive nature and the possibility of using it on humans. Since the end of the 1990s, this approach has been at the heart of research that has clarified the involvement of different structures in the decision-making process in different conditions, depending on the nature of the task, the rewards, the context, uncertainty, etc. Some teams have even tackled the structures involved in social interaction and moral judgements. The methods of investigation are all built on the same model initiated in electrophysiology by Newsome and Movshon: correlation of the BOLD signal with the choice of the subject and the task settings. The heuristic value of brain imaging methods, granted by the possibility to visualize the activated areas, making them immediately understandable by all, is an undeniable advantage of these techniques. But this advantage also has drawbacks. The spatial resolution to the order of mm^3 focuses the attention of observers on the cortex, which represents about 80 per cent of the total brain volume in humans,[5] but only 25 per cent of neurons.[6] The method thus overstates the role of this structure, which is known to appear late in phylogenesis and develops slowly in mammals. This 'cortico-centrism' cannot account for how corvids, for example—which like all birds, are equipped with a pallium, a very archaic version of the cortex—are nevertheless able to perform complex cognitive tasks including the mirror test[7] (see Chapter 2). The BOLD signal is also particularly noisy, so only a strong signal can be measured. As a result, for each task, only a small amount of brain areas 'light up'. The consequence is that, by combining these two biases, we have seen simplistic explanations, attributing a particular function to a particular cortical area, flourish. From studies whose scientific value are indisputable, a pseudoscientific vision has been developed in which the cortex has been sliced into areas of fun, choice, regret, procrastination and so on. We are not far from the glorious days of phrenology, the pseudoscience invented by Gal in the eighteenth century, which claimed to be able to predict the cognitive skills of subjects by observing the shape of their skulls.

The Tale of the Two Brains

A pernicious avatar of this neo-phrenology approach is the opposition between right brain (rational and calculator) and a left brain (intuitive and artistic). This example is one of the most prominent of many abusive generalizations of observed phenomena in the brain. That old-age favourite, fodder for staff management and personal coaches, was involuntarily originated by Fink and Marshall.[8] They used a task in which the right brain hemisphere 'lit-up' when the subjects focused on details, and the left when they focused more generally on the whole structure. This task was an example of a known fact that some areas are more specialized on one side than the other (e.g. Broca's area, which is involved in the semantic processing of language, located to the left hemisphere

[5] Swanson (1995).

[6] Twenty-one billion neurons in the cortex out of a total of 100 billion neurons throughout all the nervous system (Pakkenberg and Gundersen 1997; Pakkenberg et al. 2003).

[7] Prior et al. (2008).

[8] Fink et al. (1996).

in 80–90 per cent of the population), but it didn't imply that the dominant hemisphere works independently from the other. The fact that for some people the asymmetry is less pronounced than for others attests otherwise.[9] However, New Age psychologists have developed this idea *ad absurdum* into 'right' and 'left' personalities. Despite the fact that this myth has been contradicted several times,[10] it is still widely diffused.

Master and Servant

While functional imaging strives to highlight areas involved in the decision-making process in the cortex, electrophysiologists are interested in subcortical structures that are more developed in rodents and primates, the animal models they use. Their work shows that if one can correlate the activity of the prefrontal cortex to the choices made by animals, the same properties can be found in subcortical structures that are called basal ganglia. We'll describe these structures in more detail in Chapter 5, but it may be good to remember that they are already present in the earliest vertebrates such as the lamprey. Moreover, it is these structures that receive the greatest input of dopamine, which plays a crucial role in the learning process, as discussed in the second part of this book. This role of the basal ganglia in the learning process and decision-making is also confirmed by functional imaging studies in humans. Therefore, maintained by a certain parochialism, the debate rages between those who support the leading role of the cortex and those who defend that of the basal ganglia. It must be said that the two structures are closely interlinked and that it is probably simplistic to attribute to one of the two a necessary and sufficient role. That said, I am forced to admit that I belong to the family of electrophysiologists of the basal ganglia and so I cannot avail myself of total neutrality in the debate. I will content myself for the moment to reiterate that these structures appeared before the cortex in evolution.

[9] Zago et al. (2016).

[10] E.g. Nielsen et al. (2013). We also showed in 2009 that if a subject is involved in a One-Arm Bandit-type task which involves validating his choice by a movement of the right hand for one option or the left hand for the other, the decision results from the difference of level of activation between the left and the right orbito-frontal cortices. If his right orbitofrontal cortex prevailed, the subject pressed the left button and vice-versa. So we are indeed witnessing a clash between right brain and left brain, but to control left and right side of the body, not unlike that famous scene from Dr. Strangelove when the right hand of the eponymous character tries to strangle him while his left tries to stop him. Palminteri et al. (2009).

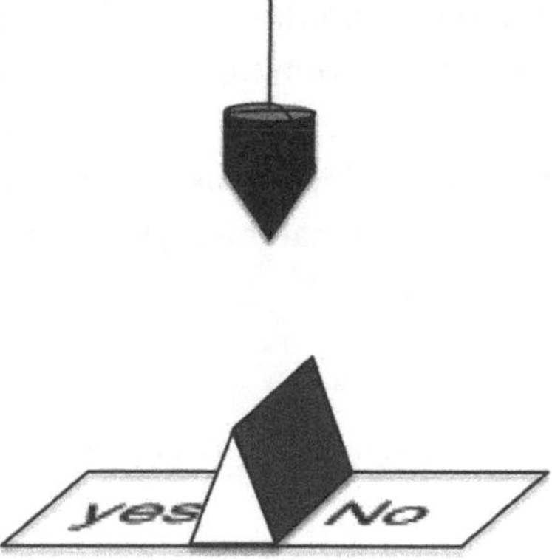

Fig. 2.2 Executive decision-maker. A pendulum is attached to a reel and is rewound with a crank. When it is released, it meets a wedge that makes it fall on 'yes' or 'no' with even chance. It symbolizes the arbitrariness of decision-making taken by the bureaucratic society described in 'Brazil'.

The Normative Approach to Decision-Making

What is decision-making in terms of the nervous system? The reader will doubtless be surprised to learn that this crucial issue is almost never discussed in publications dealing with decision-making. In the best case, as we have seen, researchers demonstrate a correlation between the activity of a neuronal population and the choice made. More generally, they identify the involved structure which then becomes a box they fit into their scheme of decision-making. The real question, 'How does the decision emerge?', is simply forgotten. It is true that there is vagueness in the definition of decision-making that does not help. We therefore must define first the meaning that we give to the term decision-making.

In order to avoid falling into the pitfalls of speculation, we use a definition that we can operationalize. We consider decision-making to be the selection (choice) of an option from several available (often two for simplicity). This definition is perfectly symbolized by the 'executive decision-maker' (see Figure 2.2), a mechanical alternative to the tossing of a coin, invented by Terry Gilliam for his film Brazil (1985). We thus free ourselves of notions of consciousness, unconscious, subconscious etc., particularly difficult to define and especially to be tested experimentally. This normative approach is close to the approach of the economists who have emancipated mentalist considerations of psychology in the twentieth century. With our decision-making being objectified by an observable behaviour, we can study it in worm, octopus, or human. Incidentally, this approach also allows us to dissociate decision-making and learning. A decision does not need to be adapted. It is independent of the result.

Learning is thus defined as a mechanism that biases decision-making. It is a dynamic process: rewarded decisions are reinforced and those that are not (or that lead to punishment) are repressed.

So now that we own a normative definition of decision-making and learning, we can address the central question of this book: How does the nervous system decide?

PART II

THE NEUROBIOLOGY OF DECISION-MAKING

3
Introduction to Information Transfer in the Nervous System

One must remember that all our temporary psychological knowledge should one day be establish in the matrix of biological substrates.[1]

Introduction

It is difficult to understand the processes described in this book without having a certain fundamental knowledge about information transfer in the nervous system. This paragraph recalls the main notions. Readers familiar with them can easily move on to the next chapter.

The Elemental Brick: The Neuron

The nervous system is organized around specialized cells called neurons, described fist by Ramon y Cajal, a great Spanish physiologist of the 19th-century, Nobel Prize of Medicine (Fig. 3.1). These neurons, which are about 100 billion in a human brain, contact each other via structures that we call synapses. Each neuron contacts an average of 10,000 other neurons.

The Action Potential, Support of Information

The neurons generate unitary electric pulses of invariant form and duration called action potentials or spikes. The quantity of spikes produced per unit of time is conventionally quantified in spike per second (spikes/s). Neurons have an intrinsic firing frequency that is their frequency of producing spikes when they are not influenced (Fig. 3.2A). We call phasic neurons those with an

[1] Sigmund Freund!

How the Brain Makes Decisions. Thomas Boraud, Oxford University Press (2020). © Oxford University Press.
DOI: 10.1093/oso/9780198824367.001.0001.

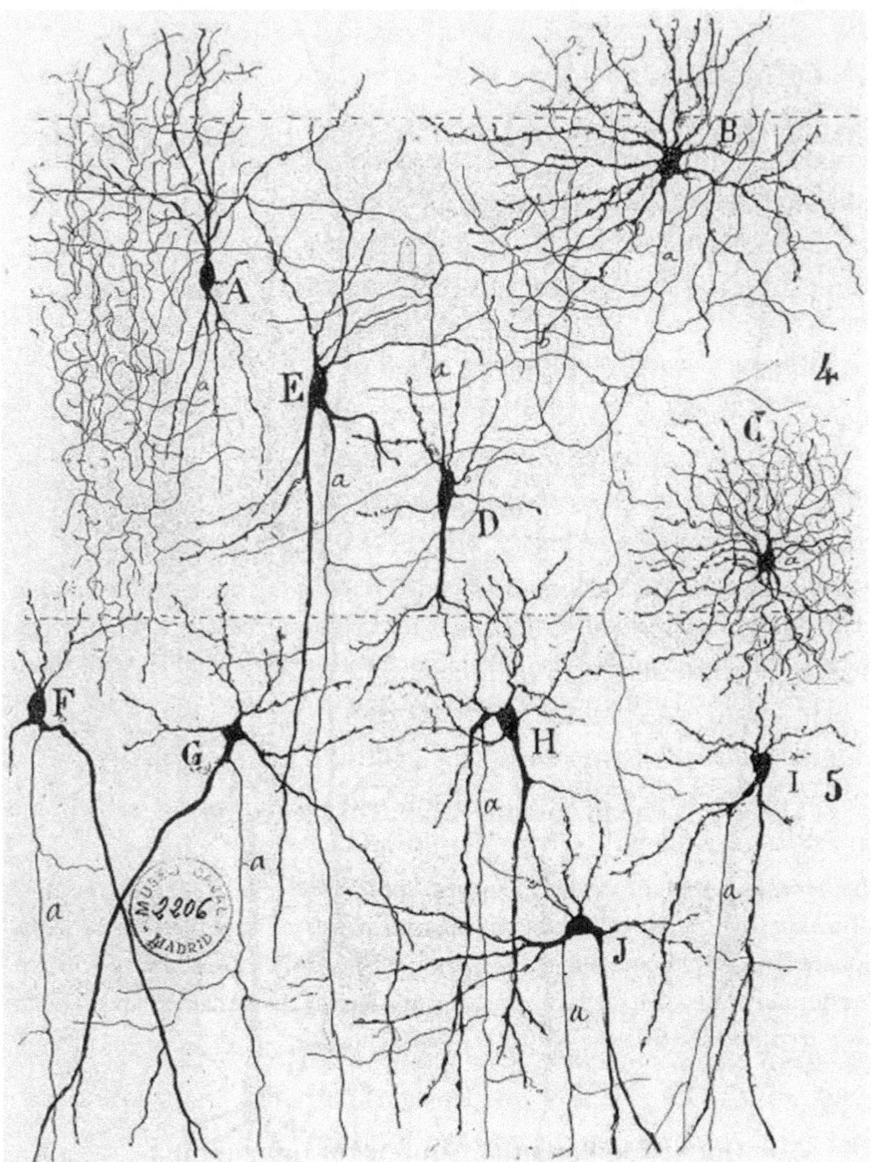

Fig. 3.1 Different neurons hand drawn by Santiago Ramon y Cajal circa 1890.

intrinsic frequency close to 0: the neuron produces action potentials only if it is subjected to an excitatory external influence. Tonic neurons have a high intrinsic activity (several tens of spikes/s).

Neurons works as integration units that transform all received information into new information. The variation of their firing frequency is constantly

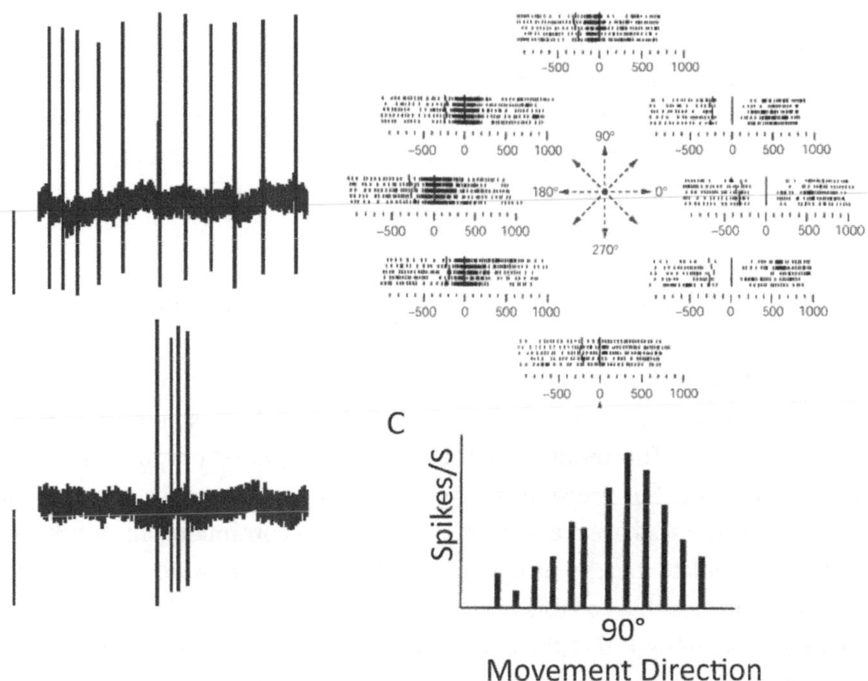

Fig. 3.2 Transfer of information into the nervous system. (A) Mode of firing of neurons. The top figure represents a tonic neuron, firing continuously and more or less regularly. The lower neuron is a phasic neuron. It produces virtually no action potentials when it is at rest, but bursts in response to a stimulus, in order to generate behaviour, etc. Of course, these are archetypes, the biological reality is usually somewhere between these two extremes. **(B and C) Information coding.** B represents the responses of a neuron in the area M1 of the primate motor cortex during the execution of a two-dimensional movement. Each group of five lines represents the response of the neuron to five repeated forearm movements in one of eight directions (0–315°) from a central position. The x axis represents time (in ms) and each vertical line represents the occurrence of a spike. The neuron increases its firing rate to the maximum when the animal performs a forearm movement to the left (180°). This direction is called the preferred direction of the neuron. Histogram C summarizes the responses for the eight directions and shows a cosine distribution around the preferential direction (we call this histogram the tuning curve of the neuron). It is thus possible to decode the information transmitted by the neuron and to infer the direction of movement performed by the animal from the firing rate encoding the information. Here the coded parameter is the direction of movement (and each neuron has its own preferential direction), but this type of coding has been demonstrated for a wide variety of motor parameters (speed, amplitude, torque), sensory (visual, olfactory, tactile, auditory) and also, as we will see, cognitive parameters depending on the area of the brain in which the recordings were made. Onset of Movement: beginning of the movement. Reproduced from Georgeopoulos et al. (1982).

regulated by the balance between the excitatory and the inhibiting inputs (see below). If the balance is in favor of the former, their activity will increase, if it is in favor of the latter, it will diminish. It is the frequency variations of these action potentials—that is, the amount of action potentials per unit of time—that convey information in the nervous system (Fig. 3.2B and C).

The Production of Spikes Is a Stochastic Process

Neurons do not produce their spikes with regularity. We are able to measure their firing rate, but we are not able to predict accurately when an action potential will occur. This results from the fact that the process of spike generation is not automatic, but probabilistic (in mathematics one speaks of stochastic process). At the scale we are interested in, time is a continuous linear process, but to manipulate it easily using a formalism derived from discrete statistics we use an artifice that consists in cutting it in time interval *t*. We can thus define the probability P that the neuron produces an action potential over this time interval *t*. For reasons that we will not discuss here, we consider that the nervous system functions on a millisecond time basis. Thus, one can describe, the behaviour of a neuron which has a discharge frequency of 10 spikes/s by the probability of producing 1 spike at each instant t=1ms that is P=0.01. This process follows a distribution law described originally by Simeon Denis Poisson[2], which is characterized by a mean equal to the variance of the distribution. It is therefore often called a Poisson process.

The Production of Action Potential, a Noisy Process

From the early age of single neuron electrophysiology, however, neurophysiologists found that even under conditions of maximum stability, the firing rate of neurons recorded *in vivo* displays variability over time. Therefore, the variance of the firing rate is generally greater than the mean in apparent violation of the law of Poisson. The difference between the theoretical variance of a Poisson process and the variance observed is usually called noise.

[2] This approximation is not fully accurate because a certain number of phenomena cause the production of action potentials to violate the Poisson process. However, we will stick to it because it is self-sufficient for our purpose and it is much more practical to describe a process with a single parameter.

For scientists who study sensory or motor processes, noise is a problem because it disrupts the reliability of the transmission of information. Some even deny the existence of noise, attributing the observed variability to our incapacity to master all the external parameters that influence the process of production of spike. On the other hand, as we shall see, with regard to the decision-making processes noise is an appreciable asset.[3]

The Chemical Synapse, Information Relay

The transfer of information from one neuron to another takes place at the synapses. There are several types of synapses, but we will only describe the chemical one that is the essential relay between two neurons. The information is only transmitted in one direction in chemical synapses. The electrical impulses of the presynaptic neuron are transformed into a chemical signal by the release of molecules called neurotransmitters into the space between the two neurons called synaptic cleft. The higher the frequency of action potentials, the greater the number of neurotransmitters released. These neurotransmitters bind to receptors on the postsynaptic neuron, where this biding produces a new electrical signal called a post-synaptic event (Fig. 3.3). This neuron sums all the post-synaptic events and that influence eventually its frequency of production of action potentials.

Synaptic coupling (or gain) is the strength of the relationship between two neurons. It determines the intensity of the postsynaptic response according to the activity of the pre-synaptic neuron. This coupling varies from one pair of neurons to another and the same neuron can be coupled differently to different target neurons. The coupling will depend on the amount of neurotransmitter released, the concentration of receptors present on the postsynaptic membrane and many molecular factors that interact with these processes and which are the subject of a very abundant literature but that we will not detail. For the same pair of neurons, this gain can vary over time this is called synaptic plasticity.

There are two major families of neurotransmitters. In general, a neuron releases only one type of neurotransmitter belonging to one of these two families.

The first family is that of excitatory neurotransmitters. The neurons that release them are naturally called excitatory neurons. When they bind with postsynaptic receptors, they have a facilitating effect on the production of

[3] Guthrie et al. (2013).

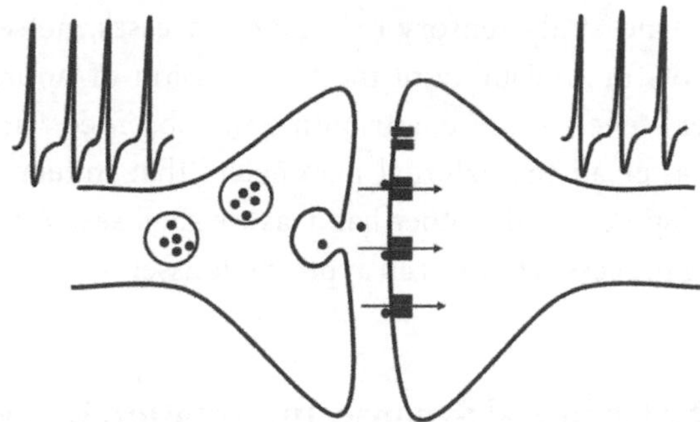

Fig. 3.3 The chemical synapse. The spike trains cause the release of neurotransmitters into the synaptic cleft. They bind to the receptors on the postsynaptic neuron. If they are excitatory neurotransmitters (glutamate, acetylcholine), they will cause electrochemical changes (by modification of transmembrane currents) on the post-synaptic neuron which will increase its production of spikes. In the case of inhibitory neurotransmitters (GABA), the postsynaptic neuron will decrease spike production. Many factors modulate these phenomena in the more or less longterm. All of these regulatory mechanisms are called neuronal plasticity.

action potentials. The most common of these in the central nervous system is glutamate.

Inhibitory neurons release neurotransmitters whose binding with postsynaptic receptors decreases the discharge frequency of the postsynaptic neuron. In the central nervous system GABA is the main representative of this family.

To be quite complete, we must mention a special family of neurotransmitters: the neuro-modulators. They interact with a very diverse set of receptors whose effects can be activation or inhibition according to their distribution and to which protein they are coupled. Dopamine and serotonin are part of this family. We will have to talk about it again.

We have summarized in this short chapter the modalities of transmission of information in the nervous system. We will now turn to the question that interests us in the next chapter: by which process will the choice emerge from the interactions between the different populations of neurons involved?

4

The Winner Takes It All

How Decisions Emerge

To decide is to act.[1]

Introduction

In this chapter, we will succinctly review the general principles that are necessary for a neural system to make decisions. A comprehensive illustration of the various principles is shown in Appendix A (the Diachetron). We will then examine how these principles are implemented in vertebrates in the following chapters.

An Effector System

As commonly stated by experimental psychologists and economists alike who study decision-making, we need to generate choice in order to overcome psychological bias (see Chapter 1). The simplest decision is that of choosing between two options.[2] We assume that we can generalize mechanisms of decision-making for more than two options from what we can observe within this framework. We thus require an experimental paradigm within which, for a given condition, the subject has to perform one of two similar actions. For this purpose, we need two populations of excitatory neurons that can act on the locomotor system in vertebrates, each allowing the execution of a specific

[1] I cannot find the origin of this sentence, popular with executive officers!

[2] Some people may consider that to decide between an action and nothing is even simpler, but in fact it does not necessarily involve the same mechanism as initiating an action while cancelling another that has been pre-selected (Eagle et al., 2008). Therefore, it is less obvious that we can generalize between one action and nothing compared to two to three to n actions. On the contrary, generalizing from two actions to three actions and n is actually less problematic (for discussion about the possibility of generalization see Chapter 22).

How the Brain Makes Decisions. Thomas Boraud, Oxford University Press (2020). © Oxford University Press.
DOI: 10.1093/oso/9780198824367.001.0001.

behaviour (such as moving the body or pointing a limb in one direction or the other). For a choice to be observable, one of these two populations should be activated, while the other should be inhibited. This implies a mechanism of competition between them.

Lateral Inhibition

Examination of the literature shows that the simplest system to obtain an imbalance between two populations of neurons subjected to the same activation consists of two interconnected populations of inhibitory neurons.[3] These two populations exert lateral inhibition on each other. As we explained in the previous chapter, a given population of neurons releases, generally, only one type of neurotransmitter. The neurons cannot be both excitatory and inhibitory. Therefore, in order to exert lateral inhibition on each other, our two populations of excitatory neurons of the effector system need to be connected to two different populations of inhibitory neurons that are reciprocally connected.

Noise

If the transmission of information were to be fully reliable, it would not be possible to obtain an imbalance within an architecture of two co-activated excitatory populations stimulating two reciprocally connected populations of inhibitory neurons. They would cancel each other out and the system would become stuck. In order for a differential response to emerge, noise is necessary. There are many sources of noise, an important one of which is Brownian motion.[4] At the molecular level, it animates the ions responsible for the variations of membrane potential. At the synaptic level, it also animates the receptors and the transmembrane molecules, inducing variability in neural transmission.

Furthermore, the release of neurotransmitters by exocytosis follows random processes: a spike will not systematically release the same number of neurotransmitters. Therefore, each neuron receives input from several thousand other neurons through several thousand synapses, whose random behaviour

[3] See Deco et al., 2009; Jovanic et al., 2016.

[4] Brownian motion is a mathematical description of the behaviour of a particle immersed in a fluid subjected to permanent shocks with the elementary particles (ion, atoms) of the surrounding fluid. This results in a seemingly random movement of the large particle, which was first described in 1827 by botanist Robert Brown inside pollen grains.

has non-linear properties that will induce a great variability of response to an identical stimulus. Synaptic noise is considered the main source of noise in the nervous systems.[5]

Positive Feedback

However, as it is, the system is relatively unstable: it can alternate from one state to another without modification of the stimulus. If the noise is too large, the divergence can also be triggered in the absence of stimulus. Stabilization is provided by another property called positive feedback. It means that each population of neurons exerts an activating influence on themselves, amplifying the effects of an imbalance between the two populations as it occurs. It remains as long as the stimulus lasts, and therefore maintains the divergence as long as necessary.

Learning Process

Within such an architecture, our system would work randomly. It would therefore not be possible to determine *a priori* which action would be chosen. However, if our choices have the potential to lead to different outcomes, this provides interesting opportunities for our system to learn how to select the best option. In order to achieve this, our system needs neural plasticity rules.

In the late 1940s, neuropsychologist Donald Hebb formulated the first plasticity rule that bears his name, and which can be summarized as follows:[6] if a neuron A is connected by a synapse to a neuron B, and the two neurons increase their activity together, then the gain of the synapse that joins them will be increased. So, when neuron A is stimulated, the response of neuron B will be amplified. It would take more than 20 years for the underlying mechanism to be demonstrated in the hippocampus by Lømo and Anderson[7] in the form of what he called long-term potentiation (LTP). This is a gradual increase in response from a post-synaptic neuron to the excitation of the pre-synaptic neuron that persists over time. Hebbian learning and LTP form the basis of learning processes in the nervous system.

[5] Calvin and Stevens (1968); Contreras et al. (1996); Kohn (1997); Nowak et al. (1997); Pare et al. (1998); Azouz and Gray (1999); Lampl et al. (1999).

[6] Hebb (1949).

[7] Anderson and Lomo (1966).

However, the simple Hebbian learning rule is not enough, because it increases synaptic coupling without any regard to the usefulness of the outcome. What we need is often referred to as a tri-component Hebbian learning rule, or more commonly, reinforcement learning. It implies that there is a third class of neurons, where firing is conditioned by the presence of reward and their effect is to modify synaptic coupling when activated, rather than altering the firing rate of the post-synaptic neuron. If we connect this population of neurons at the interface between excitatory and inhibitory neurons, when one of the two actions results in a reward, this population of neurons reinforces only the coupling between the populations of neurons corresponding to the selected action. The gain between the activated neurons will change from an average state to a high state, so that the competition will be biased toward the rewarded action.

Anti-Hebbian Learning

However, if by chance, the context changes and the action associated with a reward is reversed suddenly, the system is no longer able to readjust. For this, we must introduce a devaluation mechanism for a chosen option if it is no longer rewarded. The simplest solution would be to add a mechanism for decreasing the gain between excitatory and inhibitory neurons if an option is chosen and not rewarded. The mechanisms for this type of solution exist in nature, and are grouped under the term extinction.

Among these mechanisms, one of the best described is the mirror mechanism of LTP: long-term depression (aka Anti-Hebbian Learning), which causes two neurons that fire together, under certain conditions, to reduce their synaptic coupling.

Now that we have reviewed the general principles that are necessary for a nervous system to generate a decision, we will proceed to examine the architecture of the vertebrate brain in order to identify the associated network.

Implementation

To understand how these principles can be integrated into a model of the neural system that is able to decide between two options, I invite the curious reader to look at Appendix A (the Diachetron). This is an attempt to identify the minimal network of decision-making, in order to establish if we can find a similar architecture in the nervous system of vertebrates.

5
The Lamprey's Dilemma

Introduction

Any attempt to identify the circuits involved in the decision-making process must therefore consider the principles identified in the previous paragraph. However, we need to keep in mind that a number of generalization methods must be taken into account. Perceptual modalities in vertebrates are complex and multimodal; we seldom decide between two options, having instead much more open choices, etc. However, that being said, the six principles introduced in the previous chapter (Effector, Lateral Inhibition, Noise, Learning Process, Positive Feedback, and Anti-Hebbian Learning) constitute the lowest common denominator of neural decision-making systems that we should look at. This is the task we will initiate now. As our aim is to study these processes in humans, we will limit ourselves to vertebrates, which all share the same longitudinal organization and possess a brain and a spinal cord.

A Tripartite Brain

Let us first recap quickly on the organization of the vertebrate brain. It is made of two symmetrical hemispheres controlling the contralateral hemi-body: the motor areas of the left hemi-brain control the muscles of the right hemi-body. The brain hemisphere consists of grey matter, in which is located the cell bodies of neurons, and white matter, which corresponds to the pathways of axons connecting one brain area with another distant one, or with the spinal cord. The organization of the grey matter is based on the development of the brain during embryogenesis. It is subdivided into three major parts, derived from three different vesicles formed in the embryonic stage:

- The mesencephalon includes: i) the tectum, a sensory-motor organ; ii) the raphe nuclei involved in the regulation of many functions such as sleep, alertness, mood, and which also controls certain motor behaviours; and

How the Brain Makes Decisions. Thomas Boraud, Oxford University Press (2020). © Oxford University Press.
DOI: 10.1093/oso/9780198824367.001.0001.

iii) the tegmentum, consisting of the substantia nigra and the red nucleus which are both involved in the regulation of behaviour.

- The diencephalon includes: i) the thalamus: a large nucleus at the interface between the sensory systems and the motor systems; ii) the subthalamic nucleus that is associated with basal ganglia, to which we will come back in detail; and iii) the hypothalamus and the epiphysis, which are involved in the regulation of many hormonal functions.[1]
- The telencephalon, i.e.: i) the olfactory bulb; ii) the striatum and the pallidum (the two nuclei constitute the basal ganglia per se); iii) the pallium (aka mantle) of which, in mammals, the dorsal and lateral parts are called cortex and the ventral part hippocampus.[2]

We mentioned in the introduction that the cortex was among the serious candidates as substrates of the decision-making process in humans. However, the cortex appears late in evolution. In vertebrates other than mammals, the pallium has a simpler anatomical structure. It consists of a layer of cells sandwiched between two layers of communication fibres. Moreover, in the most archaic species, it represents less than 20 per cent of the cerebral mass and receives little or even no feedback from the subcortical structures.[3] To identify our decision-making system, we must therefore look for the structures of the central nervous system, common to all vertebrates, that could share the properties we have identified. It implies that if a common structure exists, it must necessarily belong to an archaic system common to all vertebrates. It seems thus wise to start with the most ancient of this taxon: the lamprey.

In the Beginning Was the Lamprey

The lamprey appeared about 560 million years ago. It is the most famous representative of the agnathans. It has a nervous system whose relative simplicity makes it a model of choice to study networks involved in locomotor activity. The lamprey is devoid of fins and moves by waving its body, which is composed of a series of muscle segments called myotomes. Each myotome is controlled by a couple of generators. Each element of a couple controls the motor neurons that activate the muscle fibres of one half of the myotome via

[1] Another great communication pathway between the nervous system and the body.
[2] Involved in memory and spatial navigation (see Chapter 16).
[3] Striedter (2017).

excitatory neurons whose neurotransmitter is glutamate. The two elements of a couple mutually inhibit each other via glycinergic inhibitory neurons.[4] When the muscle fibres on one side of the myotome are contracted, the opposite fibres are released. When a motor drive is sent from the reticulospinal cells into the spinal cord, a rhythmic activity is propagated in the various medullar segments with a rostro-caudal shift thereby generating a sinusoidal body motion of the animal that allows its movement in the water.

The reticulospinal neurons belong to the reticular formation located in the brainstem of the lamprey. These are organized somatotopically. If a differential stimulation is exerted on the neurons located on both sides of the reticular formation, the animal will turn toward the direction of the most important stimulation. It is thus possible to control the locomotion of the animal from this structure. In fact, these reticulospinal neurons act as the effector system defined in the previous chapter. We have thus found the first element of our elementary decision-making system; let us now look at its connections.

Apart from the peripheral input that comes back from the spinal cord, the reticular formation receives, among other things, input from the diencephalon and specifically the thalamus.[5] This structure allows interfacing between sensory stimuli (visual, auditory, olfactory) and the motor system.[6] The other very important targets of the thalamus in the lamprey are the basal ganglia.

The Basal Ganglia

The striatum and the pallidum are the basal ganglia of the telencephalon per se. The subthalamic nucleus (STN), which belongs to the diencephalon, and the substantia nigra (SN), originating from the midbrain, are anatomically associated with them. The term ended up designating the functional unit constituted by these four nuclei.

We will not detail too precisely here those nuclei whose anatomy and terminology vary from one species to another, but we will roughly describe their functional architecture based on the nomenclature used in the primate.[7] They are organized as follows (see Fig. 5.1):

[4] Glycine is the main inhibitory neurotransmitter of the spinal cord.

[5] The reticular formation also receives input from other systems such as the pallium, the tectum, and the GABAergic neurons of the basal ganglia.

[6] McClellan and Grillner (1984); Dubuc et al. (2008).

[7] Nomenclature in the lamprey is slightly different and still subject to fluctuation because its characterization is relatively recent. For simplicity, I prefer to use that of the hominids, which is better known, and which is the primary purpose of this book.

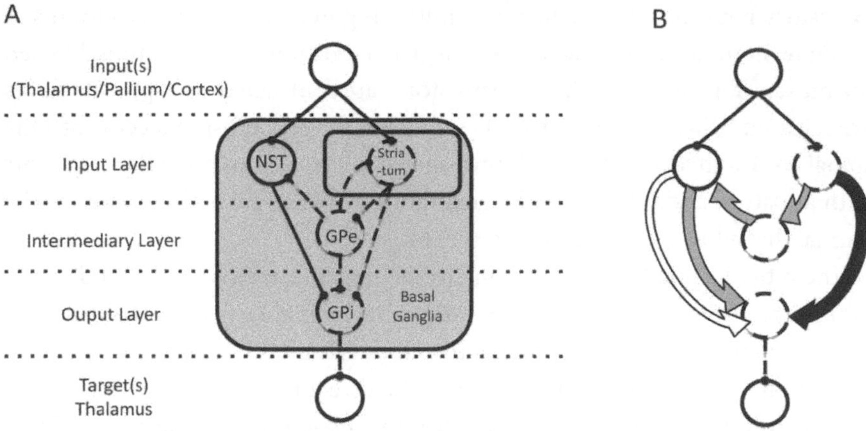

Fig. 5.1 Functional anatomy of the basal ganglia. (A) Represents the three main pathways between the input and the output structures of the basal ganglia: the direct (black), monosynaptic, indirect (grey), trisynaptic and hyperdirect (white), monosynaptic pathways. (B) The different structures are organized into an input layer, an intermediate layer, and an output layer (see the text for the abbreviations used). The neurons represented in solid lines are excitatory (glutamatergic), the neurons represented in dashed lines are inhibitory (GABAergic). In mammals, the different populations of neurons are in segregated nuclei, but in anamniotes, reptiles, and birds, they are much less well differentiated anatomically. For the sake of readability, the figure is oversimplified. For example, I have represented only the populations of neurons that connect one structure to another in mammals while there are many other populations in the striatum in particular. Also, very recent work seems to indicate that the GPe neurons that connect back to the striatum are not the same as those that connect with the STN or the GPi.

- Two input structures: the striatum and the STN;
- One output structure (sometimes subdivided into two nuclei): the internal part of the globus pallidus (GPi) in primates;[8]
- One intermediary structure: the external part of the globus pallidus (GPe).

The striatum is the most complex structure. It consists of several types of neurons; the medium-sized spiny neurons are the most numerous. They are GABAergic inhibitory neurons and their axons connect to the intermediate

[8] I am deliberately simplifying when I reduce the output structure of the basal ganglia to the GPi only. Although it is a single population of neurons in vertebrates other than mammals, in the latter, anatomically, it is divided into two structures: the GPi and the pars reticulata of the substantia nigra.

and the output neurons. These neurons are almost silent when the system is at rest and only activate when they receive many inputs.

The STN, the other input structure, has a much simpler architecture. It is a glutamatergic (excitatory) nucleus that seems to have only one population of neurons that project their axons mainly to the output structure. Whatever the species, these neurons have a tonic basal activity of a few tens of spikes.

The output structure is also made of a single population of tonic neurons with a high basal firing rate. These neurons are GABAergic (inhibitory).

The GPe, the intermediate structure, is very similar to the GPi, consisting of the same type of high frequency tonic GABAergic neurons. These neurons project their axons onto all other basal ganglia, thus exerting global inhibitory control.

If we follow the transfer of information in our mini-network of basal ganglia, we have:

- A monosynaptic pathway between one of the input structures (the striatum) and the output structure (the GPi), which has been dubbed the 'direct pathway'.
- A poly-synaptic pathway between the same two structures, which passes through the GPe and the STN, which is commonly called the 'indirect pathway'.
- And finally, a monosynaptic pathway between the second input structure: the STN and the GPi, which is called the 'hyperdirect pathway' because it is supposed to be faster than the direct pathway (see Fig. 5.1).

The pattern of the information flow in the basal ganglia has been well documented by electrophysiologists in rodents and primates in the 1990s–2000. A cortical stimulation leads to a tri-phasic response (activation/inhibition/activation) in the output structure. It has been shown, by selective inactivation of the different structures of the BG, that the early response is due to the hyperdirect pathway, the second phase to the direct pathway and the last to the indirect pathway.[9] Apart from these differences in timing and effect, the hyperdirect and the indirect pathways activate the output structure while the direct one inactivates it. Another important difference is related to connectivity (see Fig. 5.2). The direct pathway is selective: a population of striatal neurons will

[9] Deniau and Chevalier (1984, 1985); Nambu et al. (2000); Nambu et al. (2002).

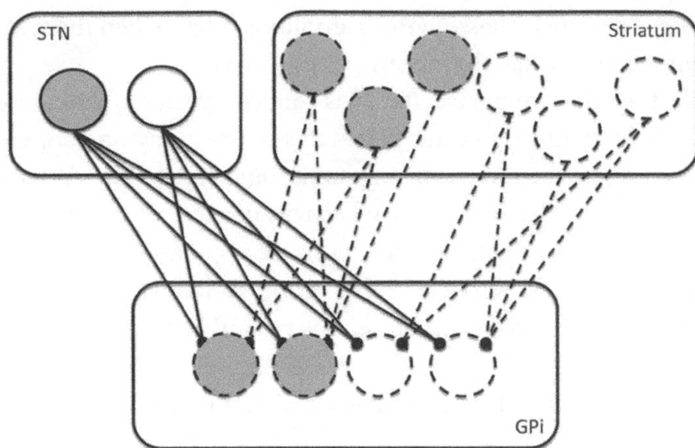

Fig. 5.2 Segregation, divergence, and convergence. The direct pathway (dotted) selectively connects the striatum to the GPi: the neurons of the grey population of the former connect with those of the grey population of the latter. It is the same for the white population. On the other hand, the hyperdirect pathway (continuous) connects the input and output populations in a sparse and nonselective diffuse manner. Note also that the number of GPi neurons (about 150.10^3 in primates) is much lower than that of the striatum (about 9.10^9 in primates), resulting in convergence. We did not represent the GPe and the hyperdirect route on this diagram for the sake of simplicity, but it is also divergent since it takes the hyperdirect route on its last third.

inhibit another GPi population preferentially and will not make connections to neurons of other populations. Conversely, along the hyperdirect pathway (and also the indirect pathway that is common with the hyperdirect pathway on its distal path), the STN neurons connect sparsely and non-selectively with the neurons of the output structure.

Thus, if we summarize, the basal ganglia constitute a network in which the dynamics result from a selective direct inhibitory pathway whose effects are in balance with the hyperdirect and indirect pathways whose effects are excitatory, sparse and non-selective. These properties have been demonstrated in mammals, but it has been shown relatively recently that this was already the case in the earliest vertebrates and has been conserved throughout evolution. It has been particularly characterized in lamprey and songbirds. In these species, macro-anatomical segregation in nuclei is not complete but the different populations of neurons coexist in poorly differentiated clusters.

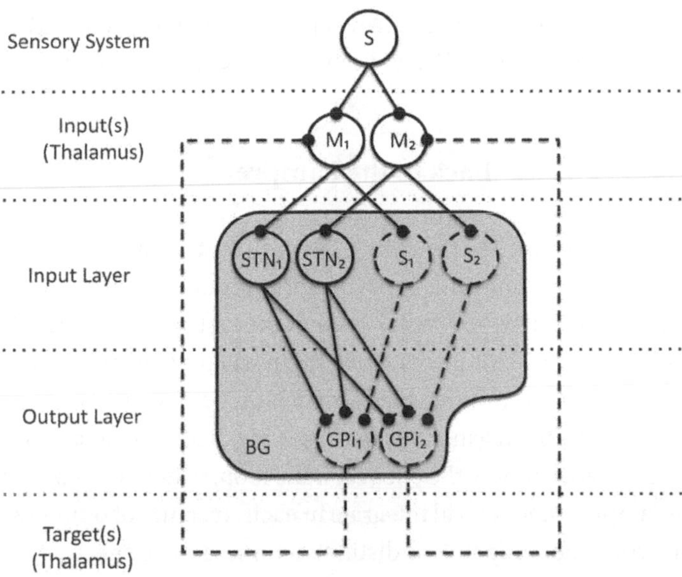

Fig. 5.3 The diencephalic network in anamniotes. The architecture of the network as it is known in lamprey is downscaled to the level of two neurons in the thalamus: M1 and M2 which each control a different action (a movement to the right for M1 and to the left for M2 for example). The corresponding actions were not represented to simplify the figure. The sensory system is reduced to its simplest expression: a neuron S connecting evenly with M1 and M2. To each of the thalamic neurons corresponds a neuron in the other structures of the loop. Note that the pathways between the striatal neurons (Str1 and Str2) and the GB output neurons (GPi1 and GPi2) are independent, while each STN neuron connects the two GP neurons according to the divergence principle (Fig. 5.4).

The Diencephalic and Telencephalic Loops

The basal ganglia fit into a functional loop. In all anamniotes, such as the lamprey, this loop is constituted mainly with the thalamus (see Fig. 5.3): the latter provides the majority of the input to the striatum and the STN and receives massive connections of the output neurons of the basal ganglia (equivalent of the GPi neurons in primates).[10] We will call this the thalamus-basal ganglia loop, the diencephalic loop.[11] There is also a pallium-thalamus-basal ganglia

[10] Reiner et al. (1998).

[11] This term is not official. It is also not completely accurate. It should be called a diencephalic-telencephalic loop because the basal ganglia are predominantly telencephalic structures. However, I will use it in this book for the sake of simplicity to avoid repeating thalamus-basal ganglia constantly.

loop, with similar organization, but which plays a negligible role in the genesis of behaviours in these species. We will call it the telencephalic loop.[12]

Back to the Lamprey

This long digression aimed to describe a network that forms a functional loop. The few readers I have not yet lost have kept in mind that in this archaic organism we have identified the effector system, the first element of our decision-making system. The most intuitive among them will probably have understood that we will now look in this network for the other elements. For this we will close the loop on the basal ganglia system (see Fig. 5.3) to form a diencephalic loop (let's leave aside for now the telencephalic loop, which, we repeat, is anecdotal in the lamprey) and we will integrate in each structure of our network two populations corresponding to two distinct actions. The connectivity between the different populations will obey the rules shown in Fig. 5.4. Finally, for the sake of simplicity, we will remove the indirect pathway because its dynamic properties are similar to that of the hyper-direct pathway in the first estimate.[13]

Following these principles, we obtain the structure represented by Fig. 5.4. We have our effector system (the M1 and M2 neurons) of the thalamus that act on the spinal cord and can control two different actions (the behavioural register of the lamprey is limited).

We will limit ourselves to determining for the moment if our system is able to decide without learning because we have not yet described the system of taking into account the consequences for our animal. It must therefore have a selection mechanism, noise to tilt the system in one direction or the other, and a positive feedback mechanism to stabilize the system in three possible states: no choice; choice of option 1; choice of option 2.

The positive feedback system is the simplest to evidence: it loops on the thalamus through the striatum and the GPi following the direct pathway. Stimulation of this pathway leads to an increase in thalamus activity (see Fig. 5.4A).

Noise is one of the specific features of the structure. The responses to different experimental conditions of these structures are notoriously noisy

[12] See note 68.

[13] See Chapter 20. For a comprehensive discussion of the reasons for this approximation see Leblois et al. (2006) and Guthrie et al. (2013).

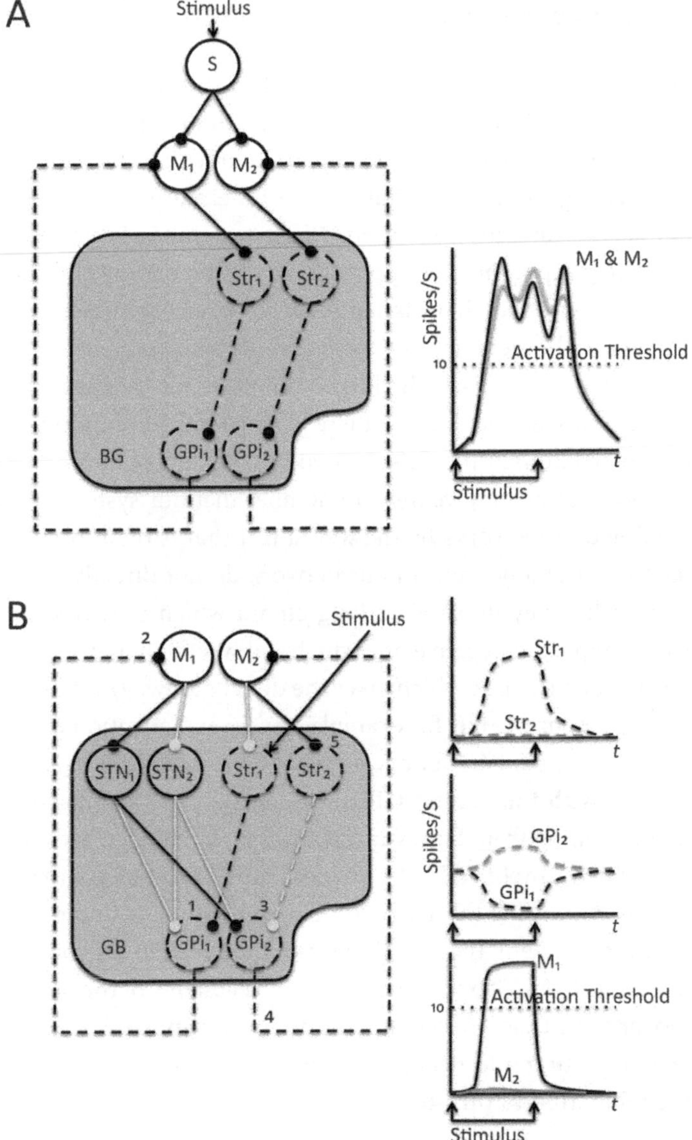

Fig. 5.4 (A) Positive feedback loop through the direct pathway. If we remove the STN and the hyperdirect pathway, a stimulation of the sensory neuron (S) leads to a significant excitation of neurons M1 (in black on the right) and M2 (in grey). Note that the presence of synaptic noise makes the excitations unstable. **(B) Competition between neurons of the striatum evidenced by a selective stimulus applied to Str1.** On the left, the connections that allowed Str1 to influence Str2 are shown in black, those non-involved are shown in grey. On the right, the firing rate of the neurons corresponding to Action 1 are in black and those corresponding to Action 2 are in grey. An excitation of the neuron Str1 causes inhibition of GPi1 (1), which increases the activity of M1 (2) and STN1. This induces an increase in the activity of GPi2 (3) that inhibits M2 (4) maintaining Str2 in an inactivated state (5). Note that the system is more stable than in the previous configuration.

and decorrelated.[14] This results in great variability in the response of a given neuron to an event (stimulus, go signal, movement initiation, etc.). This noise is amplified by a specific property of the medium spiny neurons of the striatum, which also generated an abundance of literature examining the non-linearity of the response to stimulation.[15] These neurons are particularly quiet at rest and strong input must be applied to reach their firing threshold. Once this threshold is exceeded, they discharge for a few tens of milliseconds, sometimes more, at a high frequency of several tens of spikes.

Thus, all that remains is to highlight the selection mechanism. At first sight this does not seem obvious, as there is no lateral-inhibition between the neurons of the striatum or the GPi, the two populations of inhibitory neurons in our network.[16] However, we must remember that our system operates in a loop (like all neural networks by the way, a fact that is often omitted). Thus, even if the two striatal neurons of our network do not directly inhibit themselves reciprocally, they do so via a long circuit which borrows successively from the two loops: the negative one which follows the hyper-direct pathway followed by the positive one which takes the direct pathway (see Fig. 5.4B). An activation of the neuron Str1, for example, causes an activation of the neuron NST1 which activates the inhibitory neurons GPi1 and GPi2 in an equivalent manner. But as with the neuron GPi1, this activation is counterbalanced by the inhibition coming from Str1, which causes an imbalance between the two populations which, amplified by the phenomenon of resonance that generates this loop, ends up causing the activation of one population and the inhibition of another. In this system, the selection is not produced locally by lateral inhibition, but results from interactions between all elements of the network.

Our network can thus work as a random decision-making engine (see Fig. 5.5). If we submit our model nervous system of the lamprey to a stimulus which gives it the injunction to turn to the right or to the left, the neuron S excites

[14] Nevet et al. (2007); Leblois and Perkel (2012). The electrophysiologists working on basal ganglia had a bad reputation for a long time because their recordings are notoriously noisier than those obtained in other structures such as the sensory and motor cortical areas or the hippocampus.

[15] Wilson and Groves (1981); Nisenbaum and Wilson (1995); Sandstrom and Rebec (2003).

[16] This observation has generated a huge amount of literature. Especially at the level of the striatum, which we have seen has several populations of inhibitory inter-neurons (Parent and Hazrati 1993, 1995b; Parent et al. 2000). Recent work seems to show some degree of lateral inhibition in the striatum, but it appears to be limited (Jaeger et al. 1995; Oorschot 1996; Koos et al. 2004). Some authors rely on these results to model the physiology of the network and it must be admitted that their solution has the merit of being simple and elegant (Groves 1983; Alexander and Wickens 1993; Kotter and Wickens 1995; Wickens et al. 1995; Bar-Gad and Bergman 2001; Suri et al. 2001). We prefer not to take this into account because their effectiveness is not fully demonstrated and we show that the architecture of the system is such that we can do without it (see Leblois et al. 2006 and Guthrie et al. 2013 for the demonstration). If it turns out that lateral inhibition is confirmed in the striatum then it will only strengthen the mechanisms proposed here.

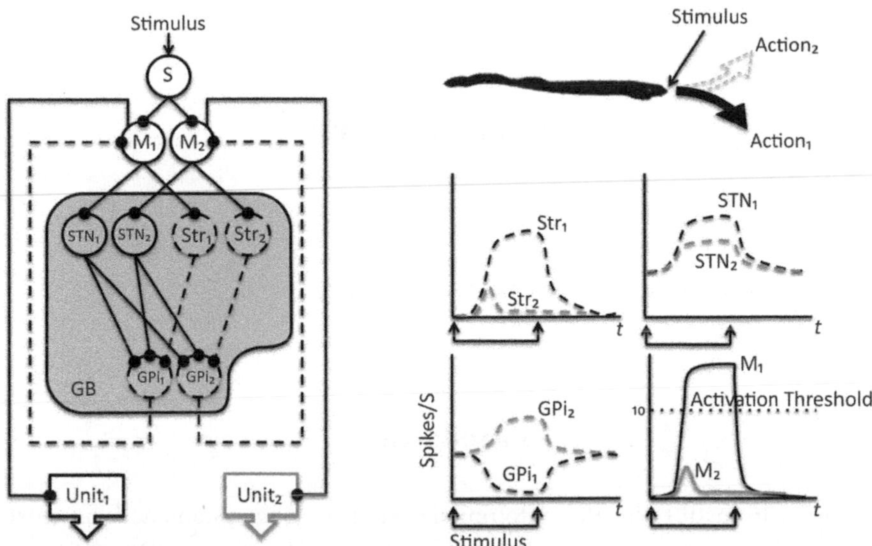

Fig. 5.5 The diencephalic network of anamniotes: a decision-making engine. When a stimulus is applied to the neuron S, the interaction between the direct and indirect pathways provides the necessary properties for one of the two actions to be chosen: a competition process between two inhibitory neurons (see Fig. 5.4B), noise, and the positive feedback amplification process (see Fig. 5.4A). For the moment, in the absence of a learning mechanism, these decisions are random. In the example shown on the right, Action 1 will be initiated thanks to the activation of the M1 neuron (in black).

M1 and M2, but the synaptic noise at the connection between the M-Str and Str-GPi neurons causes an imbalance between channel 1 and channel 2. This imbalance is amplified by the phenomena of negative and positive feedback, which selectively activate one of the two populations M. Since there are no negative or positive consequences for these actions and the system lacks a learning process, our fictional lamprey will randomly turn right or left in response to a single stimulus.

We have identified a network, already existing in the earliest vertebrates, which has the characteristics of a decision-making system. Is it capable of learning? How did it evolve? Is the neuronal structure able to solve competitions? Can it be replaced by another system during evolution? These are all fascinating questions that we will try to answer in the following chapters.

6
Learn to Earn

Le Cœur a ses raisons que la raison ne connaît pas.[1]

Introduction

In order to instil rationality into our decision-making system, actions must have meaning. Motivation is the driving force of behaviour. Why will our lamprey bother, if its choice to turn left or right has no consequences, either positive or negative? Negative consequences can be life-threatening (in which case the subject is not allowed to make mistakes) or unbearable (pain or the loss of a positive enhancer). These processes elicit mechanisms of fear and aversion that are still not very well known.[2] Moreover, pain and loss of a positive enhancer are probably underlaid by different networks. Finally, our initial interrogation concerned the lack of rationality and that negative reinforcement processes are less often faulted, in particular because they are much less studied, for obvious ethical reasons. With our approach being guided by the necessity of experimental validity, we will therefore focus on the positive consequences.

When studying the learning abilities of a subject, any beneficial consequence is called reward. This reward can be of a different nature. If the subjects are human, it is generally money, but other modalities have sometimes been tested, if only to assess whether there are several levels of classification for rewards (one for money, one for food, one for sex, etc.) or only one that would perform a collation.[3] When the subjects are animals, the reward is usually food (solid or liquid) for the sake of simplicity. Since we cannot restrain a lamprey's

[1] 'The heart has its reason which reason does not know', Blaise Pascal (Pensées 1670).

[2] The literature concerning aversive conditioning is plethoric but there is no consensus on the circuits involved and the underlying mechanisms (for review see: Delgado et al. 2008; Iordanova 2009; Tronson et al. 2012; Fernando et al. 2013; Reichelt and Lee 2013).

[3] Kable and Glimcher (2009); Sescousse et al. (2010); Wunderlich et al. (2012); Sescousse et al. (2013); Sescousse et al. (2014).

How the Brain Makes Decisions. Thomas Boraud, Oxford University Press (2020). © Oxford University Press.
DOI: 10.1093/oso/9780198824367.001.0001.

access to drinking water (even a virtual one), we will use an experimental paradigm with food as the reward.

So, let's modify our experimental protocol as follows: if our hungry lamprey chooses Action 1: it will get a piece of food; if she chooses Action 2: she will not get anything.

In order for our lamprey to learn to choose Action 1 rather than Action 2, we know that it is necessary to introduce a reinforcement learning mechanism and a system which informs the lamprey on the outcome of its choice.

Dopamine

This neuromodulator[4] comes into play and will have a major role. Dopamine is a monoamine[5] released by specific neurons whose role will be different depending on the family of receptors on which it will bind. If it binds with dopamine receptors of type 1 (D1) or type 5 (D5), it will have a facilitating effect on the synaptic transmission of these neurons. If dopamine binds to type 2 (D2), type 3 (D3), or type 4 (D4) receptors, it will have an inhibitory effect on synaptic transmission.[6]

Apart from a classical synaptic transmission, dopamine can also be sparsely released at the level of varicosities. This mode of release, called volume transmission,[7] ensures the molecule a wider diffusion in a mode similar to hormonal secretion of the paracrine type.[8] It is in this form that it played a role in the earliest stages of evolution.

Dopamine is found in all multicellular animals, even those without a nervous system such as sponge and corals.[9] In all the species in which it has been studied, it is associated with motor behaviour.[10] In organisms as rudimentary as earthworms[11] or aplysias[12] (a kind of sea slug), dopamine is involved in foraging—the search for food—one of the most basic rewards.

[4] As stated in Chapter 3, a neuromodulator is a molecule that modulates synaptic transmission between two neurons.

[5] I.e. a molecule synthesized by the chemical alteration of an essential amino acid (tyrosine for dopamine).

[6] Monsma et al. (1989); Gerfen et al. (1990); Sibley et al. (1992); Gerfen and Keefe (1994).

[7] Zoli et al. (1998); Bustos et al. (2004); Rice and Cragg (2008); Fuxe et al. (2013); Cachope and Cheer (2014).

[8] Paracrine hormonal communication is a signaling mode involving chemical messengers that act in the vicinity of the cell that synthesized them (Kanno 1977; Heitz 1979; Larsson 1980a, b; Frohman 1983).

[9] Cottrell (1967).

[10] Barron et al. (2010).

[11] Kindt et al. (2007).

[12] Nargeot et al. (1999); Nargeot and Simmers (2011); Bedecarrats et al. (2013).

In vertebrates, dopamine is associated with reinforcement learning and decision-making. In these species, there are several nuclei of dopaminergic neurons in the central nervous system, but also in the peripheral one.[13] There are even cells capable of releasing dopamine into the circulating blood, whose function is still poorly understood. However, the substantia nigra and the ventral tegmental area, the dopaminergic nucleus that will be of interest to us, are closely connected with our diencephalic and telencephalic loops.

The Substantia Nigra and Ventral Tegmental Area

The substantia nigra is a mesencephalic nucleus that owes its name (black nucleus) to its natural colour in mammals due to the presence of neuromelanin. It is subdivided into the pars reticulata (functionally associated with the GPi, see Chapter 5) and the pars compacta. The ventral tegmental area (VTA) is a neighbouring structure located more medially. The dopaminergic neurons are grouped in the substantia nigra pars compacta (SNc) and the VTA. Both structures innervate almost all the diencephalon and telencephalon, but it is the striatum that receives the most important proportion of dopaminergic input.[14] This nucleus is literally immersed in a bath of dopamine: the concentration is one hundred times greater than in any other brain structure in mammals.[15] As would be expected with such high concentrations, volume transmission is known to play a role into the striatum. It is very likely that this role is functionally different from the one played by synaptic transmission.

With regard to synaptic transmission, dopaminergic neurons connect with all striatal neuron populations, but it is with medium-sized spiny neurons (the projection neurons) that the connections are the most important and the best known. On these neurons, the dopaminergic terminations are close to the presynaptic button with which they are functionally associated.[16]

[13] Barbeau (1972); Goldberg et al. (1978); Creese et al. (1981); van Rooyen and Offermeier (1981); Berkowitz (1983); Snider and Kuchel (1983); Van Loon (1983).

[14] It is sometimes stated in the literature that the striatum receives 90 per cent of the dopamine produced in the substantia nigra, however I was unable to find the source of this assertion.

[15] Fitoussi et al. (2013). Data on lamprey are less consistent but seem to be compatible (Ryczko et al. 2013; Stephenson-Jones et al. 2013; Perez-Fernandez et al. 2014).

[16] Most of our knowledge on this matter comes from mammals and mainly concerns cortex-striatal connections because the cortex is the main input for these species (Parent and Hazrati 1993; Parent et al. 1995; Parent and Hazrati 1995b). The few elements gathered on the anamniotes (Menard and Grillner 2008; Ericsson et al. 2011; Stephenson-Jones et al. 2012; Ericsson et al. 2013; Stephenson-Jones et al. 2013) and birds (Gale and Perkel 2010) are consistent with it.

The two families of receptors (D1 and D2) are present in the structure but they seem to be expressed by different neurons. The neurons that belong to the direct pathway express mainly the D1-type receptors and those of the indirect pathway express rather the D2-type receptors.[17] The release of dopamine will thus modulate the activity of striatal neurons in both directions: facilitating it on the direct pathway and inhibiting it on the indirect pathway.

Dopamine and Learning

The effect of dopamine on synaptic transmission is evident in many physiological and pathophysiological processes, but it is the role of dopamine in learning that will hold our interest here. Neurophysiologists have been working in this area for about 40 years and dealing with substantial controversy, but a consensus seems to have emerged finally, at least for dopamine D1 receptors. Several experiments have shown that D1 antagonists suppress the long-term potentiation which is the experimental demonstration of tri-component Hebbian processes (see Chapter 4).[18] It is an indirect demonstration, but it has been reproduced often enough and by a sufficient number of teams for us to have confidence in its robustness.

So, we can assume that the binding of dopamine with D1 receptors facilitates learning and that dopamine is significantly released in the striatum of the lamprey as in all vertebrates.[19] The striatum of this animal is thus likely to process reinforcement (tri-component Hebbian) learning.

[17] The first decade of the twenty-first century degenerated into a genuine scientific warfare around the issue of the location of dopaminergic receptors and the degree of segregation between the direct and indirect pathways. Nowadays, it seems that the armistice has been signed after the total victory of the 'segregationists'. The two populations are almost completely segregated and the neurons of the direct pathway express only the D1 receptors while those of the indirect pathway express almost exclusively the D2 receptors (Surmeier et al. 1992; Le Moine and Bloch 1995; Robertson and Jian 1995; Aubert et al. 2000; Svenningsson et al. 2000; Deng et al. 2006; Bertran-Gonzalez et al. 2010; Thibault et al. 2013).

[18] Arbuthnott et al. (2000); Kerr and Wickens (2001); Centonze et al. (2003a); Centonze et al. (2003b); Ding and Perkel (2004); Lemon and Manahan-Vaughan (2006); Calabresi et al. (2007); Granado et al. (2008); Pawlak and Kerr (2008); Schotanus and Chergui (2008); Zweifel et al. (2008); Roggenhofer et al. (2010); Xu and Yao (2010); Dallerac et al. (2011); Hong and Hikosaka (2011); Ghanbarian and Motamedi (2013); Krawczyk et al. (2013); Roggenhofer et al. (2013); Huang et al. (2014); Suarez et al. (2014); Wiescholleck and Manahan-Vaughan (2014).

[19] Perez-Fernandez et al. (2014).

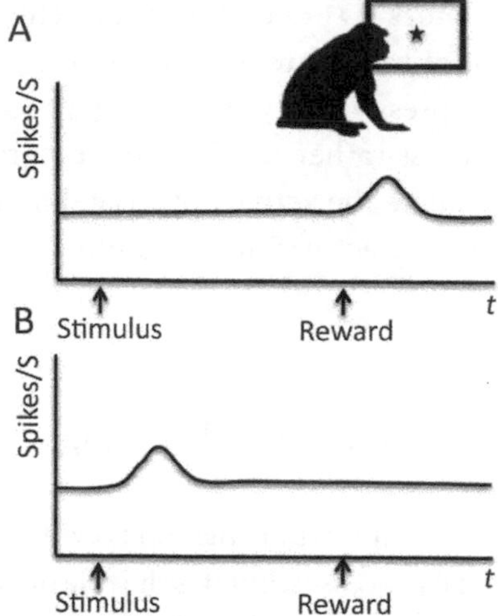

Fig. 6.1 Dopaminergic neurons and Pavlovian learning. Monkeys have been trained to focus on the appearance of visual cues on a screen. Some of these cues precede the administration of a reward (fruit juice). **(A)** At first, the dopaminergic neurons of the SNc and the VTA increase their activity in response to the administration of the reward. **(B)** Once the animals have identified which cues precede the reward, the dopaminergic neurons increase their activity in response to the appearance of this specific cue on the screen (from Schultz 1988).

Dopamine and Reward

The main reason why dopaminergic neurons interest us here is because of the relationship that binds them to the reward process. This relationship has been known since that seminal experiment which demonstrated that these neurons initially responded to reward administration, and then were able to transfer their response to the stimuli that predicted it (see Fig. 6.1).[20] Since then, the modalities of dopaminergic neurons' responses have been studied in detail and we know that their activity is much richer than a simple stimulus-response association. But for now, we will satisfy ourselves with the following approximation: when there is a reward, there is a release of dopamine.

From this, we can attribute our virtual lamprey with the following properties:

- A dopaminergic neuron that releases dopamine when rewarded.
- An increase in gain between thalamic neurons (M) and striatal neurons (Str) activated when the action performed by the animal is rewarded (reinforcement learning).

[20] Schultz (1998a).

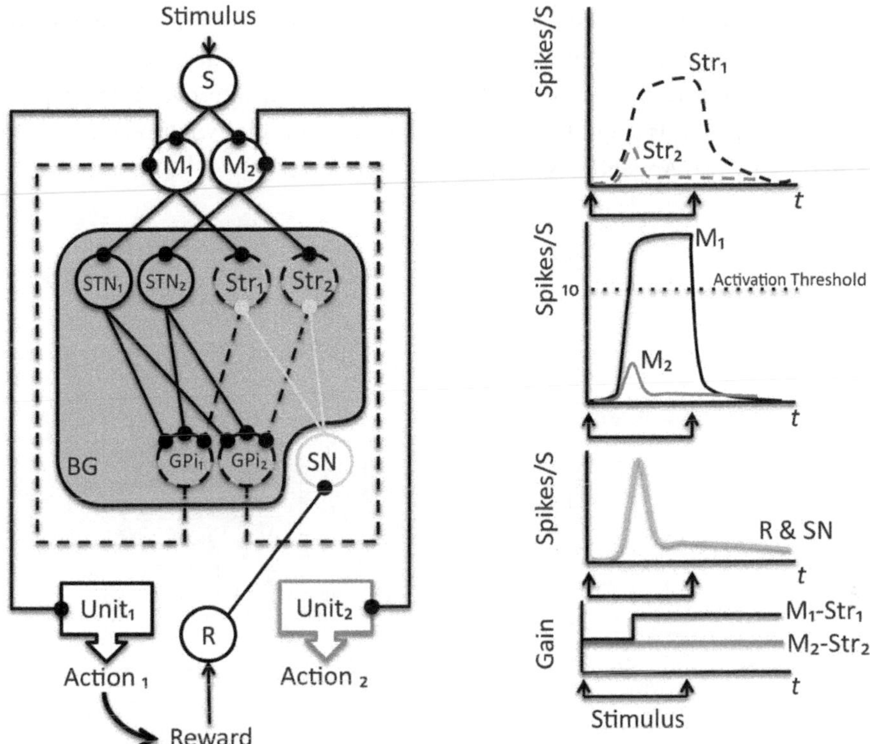

Fig. 6.2 The diencephalic network with learning capacity. We added to the diencephalic network of our lamprey a neuron sensitive to the administration of reward (R), which activates a dopaminergic neuron (with neuromodulatory properties) in the SNc. The selected action provided reward (here it is Action 1). The activation of the SNc modulatory neuron makes it possible to strengthen the gain of the M1-Str1 synapse because these two neurons are co-activated, but not that of the M2-Str2 synapse, because these two neurons have been rapidly inactivated.

- A decrease in gain between thalamic neurons (M) and striatal neurons (Str) activated when the action performed by the animal is not rewarded (anti-Hebbian learning). This last rule allows us to anticipate relearning problems or more complex tasks such as that of the two-armed bandit.

We thus obtain a neural network (see Fig. 6.2) which is now able to learn.

Exploration and Exploitation

Incidentally, if we test our neural network with a two-armed bandit task (see Chapter 1), we will observe the same behaviour as that observed first in pigeons by Herrnstein (see Fig. 1.2). This provides an anatomical substrate for the trade-off between exploratory and exploiter behaviour described by behaviourists. Therefore, one of the benefits of our bottom-up approach is to propose a robust hypothesis about the substrate that allowed this evolutionary edge to emerge (see also Appendix A for more details).

7
From Pallium to Cortex
The Coup of the Telencephalon

La fonction crée l'organe.[1]

Introduction

Nothing could be further from the truth than this maxim, which is supposed to summarize the theory of Jean-Baptiste de Lamarck (1744–1829). This French naturalist, who invented the term biology, is best known for having proposed a classification of species according to their kinship and a theory called Transformism, that states that new organs develop to adapt to changes in the environment. He was one of the influential precursors of Darwin who however moved away by proposing the theory of natural selection that overturn the view. First a mutation appears and, if it gives rise to new properties that provide an advantage over the individuals that are lacking it in the environment in which it appeared, this mutation is conserved and transmitted. The mutation eventually allows the appearance of a new species with new functions. The advent of genetics in the early twentieth century has definitely validated the theory of Darwin. If the way in which these mutations appear (gradually or by punctuated equilibrium) is still debated, the theoreticians of evolution agree on the fact that the organ precedes the function. It implies that what is conveniently called a function in biology is *de facto* an emerging property that has been preserved by the mechanisms of evolution because it provides an advantage to the organisms that possess it.

The enrichment of the ethogram,[2] a key feature in the evolution of vertebrates, is one of these evolutionary advantages. The previous two chapters

[1] 'Function creates organ.' French Lamarckian Motto of unknown origin.
[2] We define ethogram as the number and variety of individual or social behaviours that a species can display.

How the Brain Makes Decisions. Thomas Boraud, Oxford University Press (2020). © Oxford University Press.
DOI: 10.1093/oso/9780198824367.001.0001.

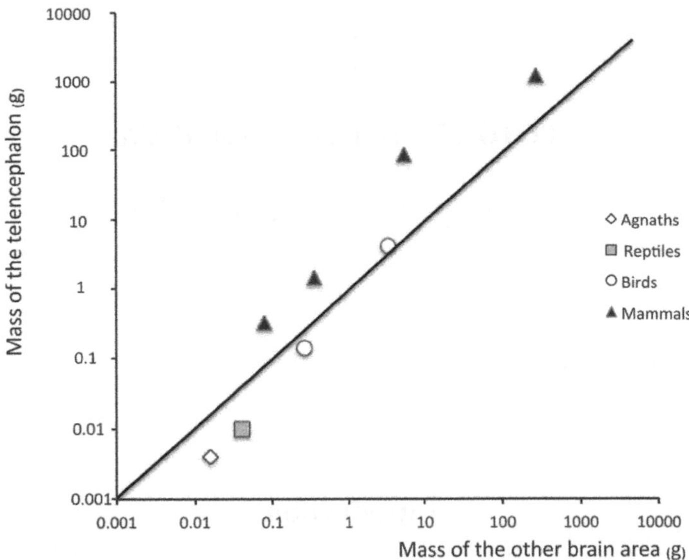

Fig. 7.1 Evolution of the mass of the pallium/cortex in the function of the mass of other brain structures (diencephalon+mesencephalon). In anamniotes, reptiles, and most birds, the telencephalon represents less than 50 per cent of the cerebral mass. In mammals, it accounts for more than 50 per cent (up to 94 per cent in some primates). Note that the scale is logarithmic.

Extrapoled from Hardman et al. (2002); Herculano-Houzel et al. (2006); Herculano-Houzel et al. (2007); Wang et al. (2007); Herculano-Houzel (2009, 2011a, 2011b); Herculano-Houzel et al. (2011); Herculano-Houzel (2012a, 2012b); Herculano-Houzel et al. (2013); Willemet (2013); Herculano-Houzel (2014). I am providing here mass and volume data, but, to be perfectly rigorous, these data should be standardized because the density of neurons does not vary in the same way in all species. For example, the neuronal density decreases with size in rodents while it remains constant in primates.

allowed us to show that the basic module of a system capable of making decisions and learning already existed in the earliest vertebrates in which the telencephalon represented less than 10 per cent of the total volume of the brain (see Fig. 7.1). The anatomy changes very marginally in other anamniotes such as fish[3] and amphibians. For all these species, the thalamus will play the role of the main relay between effector organs, which control behaviour, and sensory organs, which receive information coming from the outside environment, as in the case of our simplified lamprey (see Fig. 6.2). In fact, for these archaic vertebrates, the behavioural register varies little: foraging, mating, fight or flight reactions. Of course, there are differences from one species to another in the

[3] There is at least one exception to this assertion: some teleost fish such as Wrasses have a telencephalon that represent more than 50 per cent of the brain volume and can use tools (Bernardi 2012).

modality of foraging for example (e.g. between herbivores and carnivores), or nuptial rituals, but the whole remains largely homogeneous. The role of the diencephalic loop has been confirmed in these species with regard to eating behaviour.[4] Its role in the other behavioural registers needs to be demonstrated, but it is very likely. Reinforcement learning has been demonstrated in salamanders and newts.[5] What about other classes of vertebrates? How is their behavioural register evolving? What are the brain structures related to them?

We have, though unwillingly, a very anthropomorphic conception of evolution. Humankind, like all primates, is characterized by the development of the dorsal part of the telencephalon, which represents more than 80 per cent of total brain mass. From anamniotes to humankind, the ethogram increases in parallel to the development of this brain area; it seems natural to find a cause-and-effect relationship. Is this really the case? To verify this, let us recall the main stages in the evolution of the telencephalon in vertebrates.

The Scale and the Feather

'Reptile' is a term with fuzzy boundaries that covers several lineages of different origins distributed in more than 9,000 species, which appeared around 340 million years BC. Reptiles present a somewhat greater variety of behaviours compared to anamniotes. However, even species with a relatively high encephalization quotient (the ratio of brain weight to body weight), such as crocodiles and Komodo dragons, do not exhibit very sophisticated social behaviours. In these species the pallium represents between 10 per cent and 20 per cent of the total cerebral mass (see Fig. 7.1).

Things are changing more dramatically with birds that appeared only 150 million years ago. Although all birds are descended from a common ancestor, the 10,000+ species of existing birds have a very wide diversity of behaviour. It is in social behaviour that diversity is most apparent, such as courtship behaviours that can follow very different modalities such as singing or complex gestures but also communication about territorial issues, defence against predators, or foraging. Many bird species are organized into social groups whose complexity is comparable to that of mammals.[6] Some bird species have also developed cognitive abilities, (remember that the task of the two-armed bandits

[4] Reiner et al. (1998); Stephenson-Jones et al. (2013).

[5] Shibasaki and Ishida (2012); Retailleau et al. (submitted).

[6] E.g. the emperor penguins of the Antarctic, whose social organization was featured by Luc Jacquet in the world-acclaimed documentary 'March of the Penguins' (2004).

was developed in pigeons, see Chapter 3). The all-round champion of cognition in birds, however, is the corvid. Caledonian crows, for example, are able to use tools: they cut rods to the right dimensions to dislodge insects from their nest.[7] They are also capable of the same level of abstraction as a seven-year-old child, demonstrated through solving a task that involves throwing pebbles into a beaker to raise the water level to recover food that floats in the water out of reach of their beak.[8] Few mammals can do this.

The learning ability of birds is also well known. In songbirds such as the canary or the zebra finch, the offspring learn a song by trial and error through imitation of an adult.[9]

This enrichment of the unprecedented behavioural register is correlated with morphological and functional modifications of the encephalon of birds. Firstly, the birds generally have a higher encephalization quotient than anamniotes and reptiles. But it is the development of the pallium especially which is remarkable in these species. It accounts for more than 30 per cent of brain mass and can exceed 50 per cent in corvids (57 per cent in New Caledonian crows) and some songbirds. Although no comprehensive studies have been conducted in birds, there appears to be a strong correlation between pallium development and that of social behaviours and cognitive abilities.[10]

Cortex, Play, and Mind

Mammals appeared around 220 million years BC. The 5,400+ species of this taxon colonized from deep sea to land and air. Their behavioural register is richer and more varied than that of birds. Two behavioural characteristics, related to each other, distinguish them from other vertebrates. The first is a period of dependence of infant mammals that can last several years. The second is play.[11] During the juvenile period, much of the time saved from foraging is used to play. Although the function of this activity is still debated, it is certain that it plays a central role in the learning of foraging and social behaviours. There is, moreover, a correlation between the complexity of the social

[7] Emery (2006).
[8] Logan et al. (2014)
[9] Nottebohm et al. (1990); Mooney (1995); Tchernichovski and Marcus (2014).
[10] Cnotka et al. (2008); Herculano-Houzel (2011a); Willemet (2013).
[11] In fact, play is not unique to mammals: it has been observed in turtles and crows for example, but these are exceptions, whereas it is the rule in mammals (Bekoff and Byers 1998). It is probably not a coincidence that non-mammal species in which play is observed have a large pallium also.

organization of a species, the duration of the juvenile period, and the amount of time spent playing.

Another characteristic that is almost exclusive to mammals is the ability to recognize oneself. Of the seven species in which this ability has been demonstrated using the mirror test, six are mammals (the exception being magpies).[12]

These specific behavioural features are correlated with a general increase in the encephalization quotient and also the ratio between the size of the telencephalon and the rest of the brain. The latter already accounts for 77 per cent of brain mass in mice[13] and up to 94 per cent in some primates.[14] There is also a link between these two parameters and social complexity on the one hand versus time spent playing that evolve in parallel. Moreover, the species in which self-recognition has been demonstrated are those with the most developed telencephalon.

However, the mammalian cortex is not merely an expansion of the pallium of lower vertebrates. It is characterized by a significant structural change. The pallium consists of two or three types of neurons organized into three layers, while the cortex is subdivided into six layers of neurons and comprises 12+ different types of neurons. They are organized in a modular fashion into mini functional units organized around an output neuron. This functional unit, called a column, provides much more complex and powerful basic modules than the archaic three-layer system.[15] The richness of the ethogram of mammals is probably as much a result of this complexification as the simple increase in brain volume.

Language, Planning, and Consciousness

Man being the measure of all things, as Protagoras liked to say, it seems justified to focus on this special mammal.

Humans have long been believed to be unique, endowed with specific abilities that have classified them outside of the animal kingdom. The advent of

[12] See Chapters 1 and 11. Doubt persists for crows and some species of parrots.

[13] This ratio does not explain everything: mice have a behavioural register much more limited than that of New-Caledonian crows (mice are far from being able to use tools). It's true that the brain of a raven weighs almost 20 times more (7.5g) than that of a mouse (0.4g).

[14] Curiously, in men, this ratio is only 84 per cent, but it is true that the latter is largely offset by a massive increase in brain mass (1500g against 85g in the macaque). The decrease in the ratio is related to the increase in the mass of communication fibres between the different structures and therefore the complexity of the structure (this factor may also partly account for the paradoxical differences in ratios between the raven and the mouse).

[15] Shepherd (2011).

evolutionary theories has brought humankind back to its true place. What characterizes humanity on the behavioural level is the synergistic extension of several capacities already in existence at the embryonic stage in other species.[16] The extension of these capacities is associated with a high encephalization quotient and a cortex/brain mass ratio of around 85 per cent. The most developed cortical territory is its anterior cortex, particularly the orbito-frontal and prefrontal areas.

Amongst humanity's unique capacities, the most obvious is spoken symbolic language associated with the manipulation of abstract concepts. This ability develops along with several cortical structures, the most important of which is Broca's area (for language production), located in the left frontal cortex in 90 per cent of right-handed people, and 70–80 per cent of left-handed people, and Wernicke's area (associated with understanding), located in the left associative cortex with the same ratio. Language can be taught in a rudimentary way to some other species but homo sapiens is the only genus in which it has appeared spontaneously.

Another important skill is the ability to anticipate. This capability provides, amongst other things, the possibility of foreseeing the consequences of one's actions. This is a considerable evolutionary advantage, since it enables humankind both to i) reject a certain number of particularly disadvantageous (even dangerous) situations without having to test them, and ii) to plan a series of sequential acts whose consequences are not immediate, thus making the most of the present environment. Certain mammals (especially primates) and also crows are capable of a certain degree of anticipation but this is far below adult human capacities. It has been very clearly demonstrated that this capacity is related to the development of the prefrontal cortex and the orbito-frontal cortex.[17]

The third ability is more complex to define. It concerns what is commonly called consciousness. If we define the latter as the capacity to subjectively apprehend our own existence, it is shared with a certain number of animals of which we have already spoken. However, we intuitively feel that in humans the definition of consciousness covers a somewhat more complex reality including affective and mental states as well as a temporal dimension. These concepts are impossible to communicate without abstract language and therefore it seems unlikely that we could access them in other species even if they experienced them.

[16] Herculano-Houzel (2009, 2012b).

[17] Mackintosh (1974); Bouton (2007).

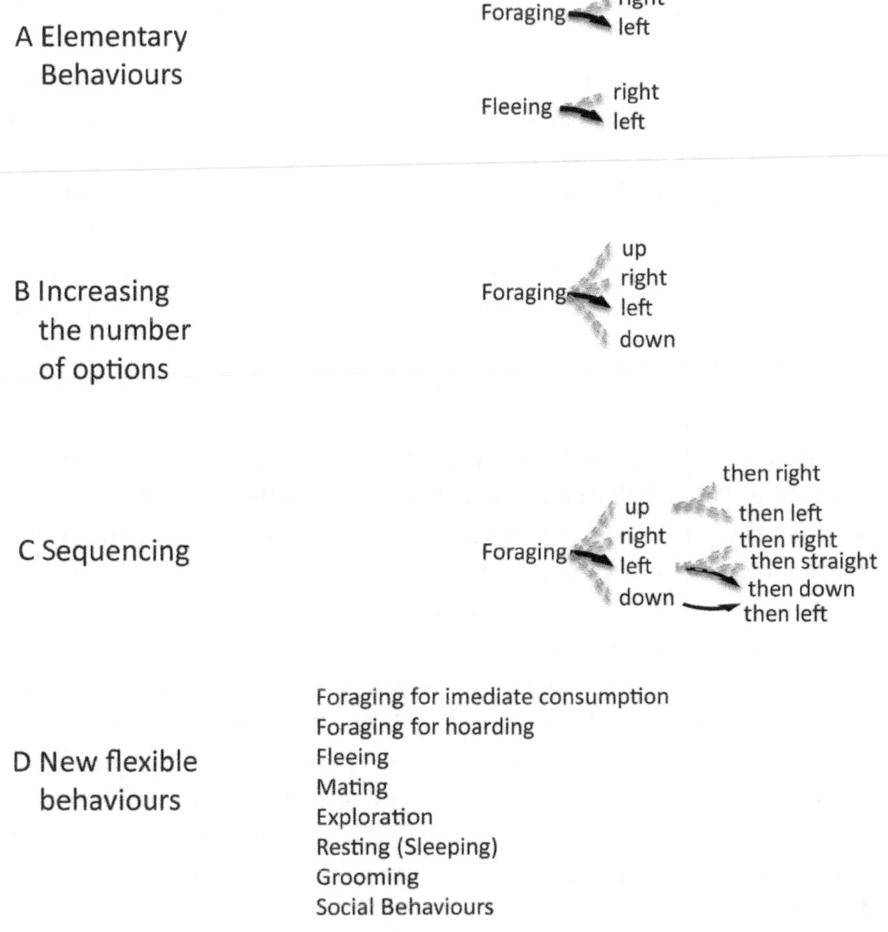

Fig. 7.2 **(A)** Several processes contribute to the increase of the register of elementary behaviours; **(B)** The increase of the number of options for a basic behaviour; **(C)** The division of the possible options into sequences; **(D)** The adoption of new flexible behaviours.

Cognitive scientists have addressed the notion of consciousness through theory of mind, i.e. the ability to decode the behaviour of other individuals. It is based on the possibility of inferring mental states: motivations, emotions, beliefs in others. It can be subdivided into several aspects: i) understanding the intentions of others; ii) understanding the perception of others; and iii) understanding the knowledge of others. Some apes, especially chimpanzees, seem to be able to infer the intentions and perceptions of others. However, no other animal except humankind appears to be able to apprehend the knowledge of others. To assess this ability, cognitive scientists use experiments that make it possible to attribute false beliefs to an individual. The best known of these experiments is that where the subject is told the story of Maxi and his mother who are in their kitchen and store some chocolate in the fridge. Then, Maxi goes to join his friends to play. During his absence, his mother decides to make a cake. She takes the chocolate from the fridge, uses some of it, and puts the rest of the chocolate in the cupboard. Later, Maxi comes back, he wants to eat chocolate. Then the subject is asked, 'Where will Maxi look for the chocolate?' The correct answer is given by children aged three to five years old. Despite the development of several equivalent nonverbal paradigms,[18] chimpanzees, who are the only animals that have been tested on this type of task, have not been able to pass this test.

This chapter affirms that there is indeed a correlation between the development of the telencephalon and the complexification of the behavioural register. However, there is no evidence that the cortex plays a determining role in the decision-making process itself. Indeed, organisms that do not have a cortex (such as newts or pigeons) are quite able to make decisions as we have defined them above (choosing between two options). They are also capable of learning and do not show a greater lack of rationality than the most advanced mammals in 'two-armed bandit' tasks (see Chapter 1). Thus, we can state that to make a decision does not require a cortex. What this really highlights is a greater diversity in the scope of the decision-making process, not necessarily an improvement to the decision-making engine itself. This diversity can be expressed in several ways: by increasing the number of available options, or a sequential division of possible responses, which thus offers a decision-making tree that further multiplies these options, or creates new flexible behaviours in the application of decision-making (see Fig. 7.2).

[18] Call and Tomasello (2008).

8
The Eminence Grise

There was Father Joseph (. . .); but his name was never mentioned (. . .) so great was the terror that inspired the Eminence Grise, the shadow of the Cardinal.[1]

Spoilt for Choice

In order for the exponential increase in the behavioural register, related to the development of the telencephalon, to benefit the decision-making process, the network involved must develop accordingly.

In the lamprey, the decision-making network is the diencephalic loop. The connections between the embryonic pallium of this species and the basal ganglia are almost negligible. It is the same with anamniotes and reptiles (see Fig. 8.1C). By contrast, the development of the pallium in birds is correlated with the development of the telencephalic loop which now supports a much larger part of the ethogram (see Fig. 8.1B). The relative ratio of flexible behaviour supported by each loop is correlated with the development of the pallium, which is highly variable in birds (20 per cent of the brain mass in hummingbirds, more than 50 per cent of the brain mass in corvids). It has been shown that in these species the diencephalic loop controls eating behaviours and also, perhaps, flying and fleeing behaviours. The telencephalic loop is involved in social behaviour—especially singing in songbirds—and cognitive processes that can be very complex, such as those in the New Caledonian crow.

In mammals, the telencephalic loop, in which the cortex now replaces the pallium, takes a leading role in controlling behaviour. The diencephalic loop alone is involved in visuo-motor coordination and hearing (see Fig. 8.1A).

[1] Translated from *The Three Musketeers* (Dumas). Father Joseph was Cardinal Richelieu's hidden adviser. He was influential in the last phase of the thirteen-years' war, triggering the intervention of Gustavus Adolphus of Sweden. Now his nickname designates those who operate 'behind the scenes'.

How the Brain Makes Decisions. Thomas Boraud, Oxford University Press (2020). © Oxford University Press.
DOI: 10.1093/oso/9780198824367.001.0001.

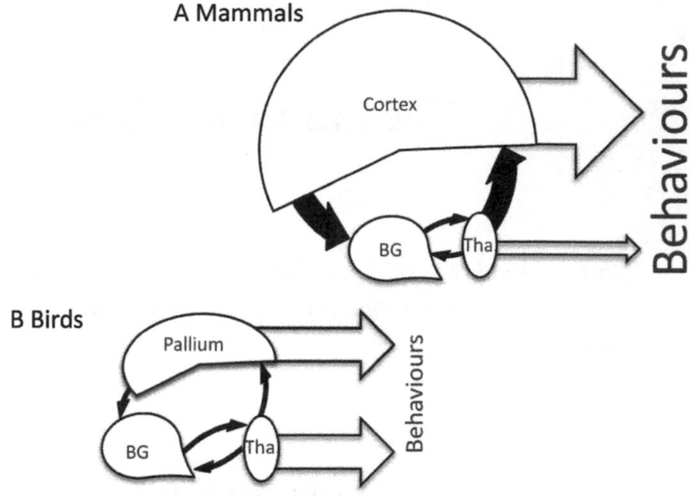

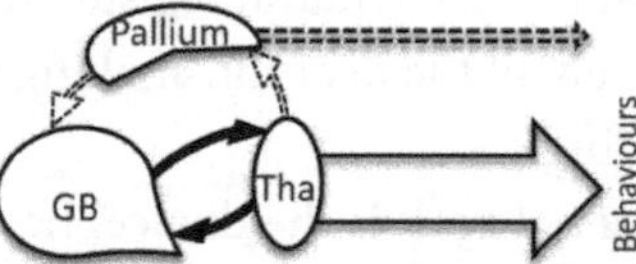

Fig. 8.1 Interactions between the basal ganglia (BG) and the telencephalon are proportional to the role of the latter in controlling behaviour. (A) In mammals, the cortex takes control of most of the behaviours in correlation with the increase in size. It also becomes the main source of input and output of the BG. (B) In birds, a transition is observed: the pallium supports a more and more important part of the behaviour (the song for example) and the BGs interact in identical proportions with the other two structures. (C) In anamniotes and reptiles, the behaviour is controlled mainly by the thalamus which is the main partner of the BG.

Thus the telencephalon, a very minor input of the basal ganglia in anamniots, gradually becomes the main input as evolution progresses.

Through the Looking-Glass

In 1986, Hershberger designed an experience he dubbed 'The room through the looking-glass', in tribute to Lewis Carroll.[2] It consisted of placing chickens

[2] I owe this reference to Dayan et al. (2006).

in a straight runway in which a feeder was set on a carriage placed on rails. The feeder moved in the same direction as the chicken, but at twice the speed. Thus, in order to have access to the food, the chickens had to learn to 'walk the other way'. Whatever the duration of the apprenticeship, the poor chickens persisted in pursuing the feeder, which escaped them continuously.

This experience illustrates *ad absurdum* what the cortex brings to the network of the decision-making process. Chickens with a poorly developed pallium are not able to act against their instinct that drives them towards food.

In contrast, primates are able to project themselves through the looking-glass. Rhesus macaques are able to perform visuospatial transformation tasks in which the relationship between the movement of a cursor on a screen is abruptly reversed compared to the movement of the joystick they handle.[3] They only need a short adaptation period of a few tens of tests to learn how to modify the movements of the joystick so that the cursor follows new trajectories imposed on them. This adaptation is correlated with a shaping of the tuning curve (see Fig. 3.1) of the neurons of the primary motor cortex. Thus, the development and complexification of the cortex not only makes it possible to increase the ethogram of mammals, but also to improve their learning capacity.

The Architecture of the Telencephalic Loop

The organization of the telencephalic loop is very similar to that of the diencephalic loop, though a little more complex. Let us describe it very briefly in primates from whom we borrowed the nomenclature of the basal ganglia in Chapter 5 (see also Fig. 8.2). Pyramidal neurons from layers three and five of the cortex provide input to the basal ganglia (striatum and subthalamic nucleus). Almost all cortical areas project onto the striatum,[4] but only the frontal areas project onto the subthalamic nucleus.[5] The feedback to the cortex is through the thalamus, whose anterior nuclei now connect extensively with the anterior cortical areas.

A quick comparison of Figs. 6.2 and 8.2 confirms that, despite a slight complexification, the main principles of selection through competition mechanisms are preserved. We still have an effector system (MC neurons), a system that initiates the behaviour (Str neuron), a mechanism of competition between

[3] E.g. Paz et al. (2003).
[4] Parent and Hazrati (1995b).
[5] Parent et al. (1989); Parent and Hazrati (1995a).

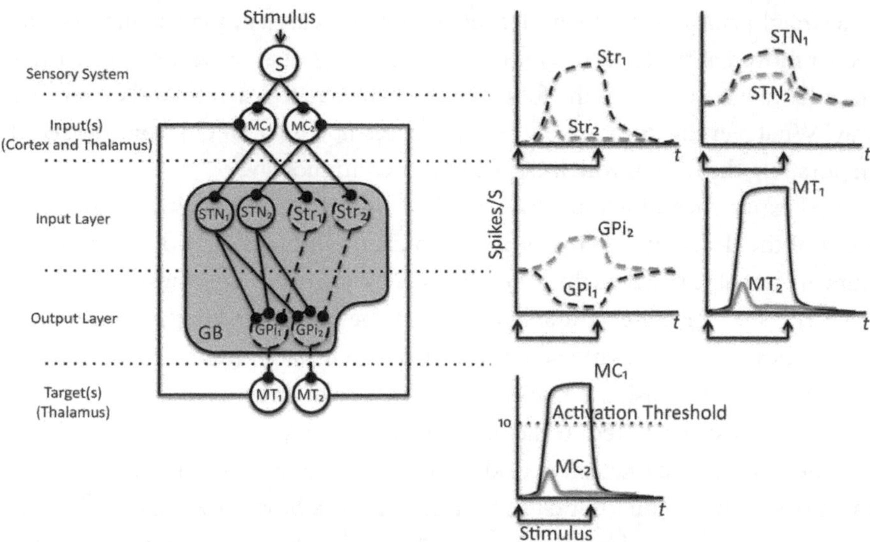

Fig. 8.2 The telencephalic network in mammals. The architecture is slightly more complex than that of the diencephalic network (see Fig. 6.2) since it adds an additional layer by subdividing the population M. Cortical neurons (MC1 and MC2) are, at the same time, the main input of the basal ganglia (BG) and the motor centres; it can be the motor cortex if the actions are movements. The thalamic neurons (MT1 and MT2) play only a role of relay between the GPi and the cortical neurons. The corresponding actions were not represented here for clarity. Since thalamic neurons are excitatory (glutamatergic) and the rest of the connections have not changed, this network has the same dynamic properties as the diencephalic network. Adapted from Leblois et al. (2006); Guthrie et al. (2013).

the inhibitory feedback loop (MC-STN-GPi-MT-MC loops), and a positive feedback mechanism that stabilizes the system in three possible states (MC-Str-GPi-MT-MC loops). The mechanism of noise generation remains the same as for the diencephalic loop.

The development of the telencephalic layer is superimposed on primitive mechanisms without modifying their intrinsic dynamic properties. This integration with an already existing system is made possible thanks to the development of the system itself. The volume of the basal ganglia evolves too, even if it is not in the same proportions as the cortex. But, and this is often ignored, communication channels also evolve accordingly. The development of the telencephalon is correlated with that of the internal capsule, the entanglement of fibres of connection between the cortical areas and the subcortical and medullary structures. It is also the conjunction of these two phenomena that explains the decrease in the ratio between the mass of the telencephalon and that of the other cortical structures in apes: the macaque has a proportionately larger cortex (94 per cent of the cerebral mass) compared to humankind (only 84 per cent of the cerebral mass) due to the fact that humankind has (a little) bigger basal ganglia and more connections.

Thus, the development of the ethogram results from the re-use of archaic processes applied to new behavioural fields: exploration, social interactions, storage of food, etc. However, the limits of these mechanisms remain the same and will be considered in the third part of this book, where we will examine the causes of the limits of rationality, which were at the origin of our questioning on these processes.

Cortical Learning

The anatomical architecture of the mammal cortex is organized in columns that enable it to perform lateral inhibition and positive feedback. The cortex is therefore also able to perform competition unlike the early pallium of the lamprey (see Figs. 8.3A,B). [6] Moreover, classical Hebbian learning (see Chapter 4) or reinforcement learning has been evidenced at the cortical level also.[7] Indeed, there is a significant release of dopamine in the cortex,[8] even if it is about a hundred times less important than in the striatum (see Chapter 6). A two-speed system is therefore possible (Figs. 8.3C,D). Initially the telencephalic loop, whose dynamics are unstable and fast, allows learning processes to modify the equilibrium of the interactions between the different cortical columns (Fig. 8.3E). Once an imbalance is established in favour of one of the columns, the cortex can take over. It would then be a consolidation process similar to the model that has been proposed for memory in which the neuronal assemblies that underlie the mental representations emerge in the hippocampus at first, then crystallize into associated cortical areas.[9] The cortex could then potentially decide alone if it was deprived of subcortical afferents (Fig. 8.3F).

Recent data confirm this hypothesis.[10] Primates were trained to choose between two targets by pointing. During the same session they were presented

[6] See Chapter 7; Shepherd (2011).
[7] Horvitz (2000); Del Arco and Mora (2009).
[8] Sesack et al. (1998)
[9] Lesburgueres and Bontempi (2011); Lesburgueres et al. (2011).
[10] Piron et al. (2016).

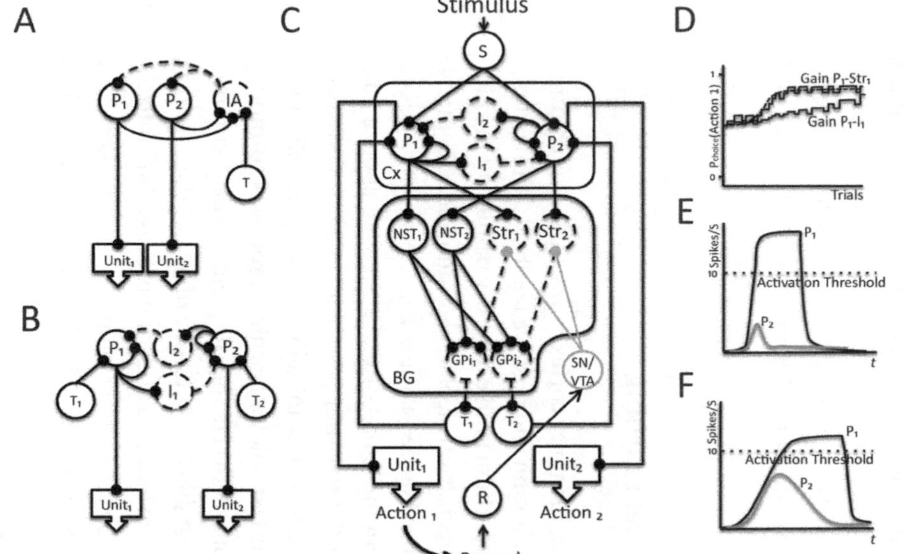

Fig. 8.3 Development of the cortex and cortical learning. (A) Model of the architecture of the pallium in anamniotes (see Chapter 7). Each module consists of only one pyramidal neuron (P). Their activity is controlled by inhibitory inter-neurons (IA, there are several types, but here they are simplified into a single population). The thalamic neurons connect with IA. This system does not have the capacity to perform selective activation of one of its modules by itself. (B) The architecture of the cortex is more complex. It is organized into columns consisting of several inter-neurons around an output. For the sake of simplicity, a column is reduced here to a module consisting of two neurons: a pyramidal neuron (P) and an inhibitory neuron (I). Only noise is missing for the system to be able to diverge (see Appendix A). (C) The cortical compartment is inserted into our previous model (see Fig. 6.2). (D) Dopaminergic neurons from the subtantia nigra (SN) and ventral tegmental area (VTA) alter cortico-striatal (P-Str) and cortico-cortical (P-I) gains. The rate of P-I learning enhancement is much slower than that of P-Str gains. (E) After learning, the dynamics of divergence between the activity of neuron P1 and neuron P2 (in the case where it is Action 1 that is rewarded) remain identical to that of our previous model. (F) On the other hand, if one removes this feedback after the cortical learning is established, the system reduced to the cortical circuit is now able to diverge (thus to choose between Action 1 and Action 2), but with a slower rate.

alternately with pairs of targets they were familiar with, followed by pairs of targets they were unfamiliar with. These targets were associated with different reward probabilities (0.25 and 0.75 in both cases), so that there was always a better choice regardless of the condition. When the familiar targets were presented, the animals preferentially chose the one associated with the highest utility (i.e. the one with an associated reward probability of 0.75). When new targets were presented they chose at random first and then, after completing a few dozen trials, they began to prefer non-exclusively the target of greater utility. Blocking the operation of the telencephalic loop through the pharmacological inhibition of GPi neurons does not alter the performance of animals when they have to choose between known targets. On the other hand, it causes an inability to choose between two new targets: the animals continue to select them at random. Another interesting aspect of this experiment was that the reaction time of the animals lengthened in both cases. This confirmed that in primates, after learning, the cortex can do without the basal ganglia when making a decision, but this takes longer.

The presence of the cortex does not alter drastically what we have discussed about the telencephalic loop, but it does open up interesting questions: Is this the case in all mammals or does it specifically relate to primates?[11] Is this the case for all cortical areas or only certain ones?

From the Evolution of Species to Neural Darwinism

At this point, it may be necessary to summarize this part of the book for the reader lost by the density of the concepts exposed. After defining what we mean by decision-making and learning, we have shown that what we call rationality results from the conjunction of these two processes. Then we demonstrated what deciding implied in terms of neuronal processes (activation of certain populations and repression of others). We then identified the basic principles necessary for decision-making to emerge in a neural network. These principles involve competition mechanisms (which require negative feedback loops), stabilization processes, and random noise. Learning is made possible by phenomena of plasticity that can bias the choice of a subject to the most interesting option. We then went on to illustrate that these principles are united in a network present in all vertebrates

[11] In rodents, it appears that the inactivation of the striatum impairs the capacity to choose between learned options (Gage et al. 2010).

since the most ancient, which we have called the diencephalic loop. This loop consists of the thalamus and a heterogeneous structure called the basal ganglia. Dopamine controls the plasticity of the network and thus enables its learning capacities, limited by the constraints of the network (presence of noise, necessity to choose initially and then to be able to switch preferences in case of modification of the context but limiting the possibility of optimizing). In the chapters that followed, we recalled that the evolution of vertebrates resulted in the development of their behavioural register and of the mantle of their telencephalon (called the cortex in mammals and the pallium in other vertebrates). This resulted in the development of a telencephalic loop, which exists only in a rudimentary state in anamniots. It has a structure very similar to the diencephalic loop and operates on similar principles. It shares the same mechanisms and limitations.

If we reframe this in an evolutionary perspective, we can assume that evolution in vertebrates is based on the explosion of the ethogram underlied by the recycling of the system of selection and learning initially devoted to locomotion and eating behaviours. In the eighties, Jean-Pierre Changeux and Gerald Edelman (both neurophysiologists), and Alain Connes (a mathematician) proposed the concept of Neural Darwinism to explain the mechanisms implemented in the brain. Through a process of '*mise en abîme*', they stipulated that the same two processes, whose conjunction was the driving force that presided over evolution at the macroscopic level, were also at work anatomically and functionally in our nervous system. These two processes were: i) a diversity generator, which offered a number of options, and ii) a selection mechanism which allowed the selection of options that were most appropriate to the situation from a panel of options. At the macroscopic level, the mutations fulfilled the role of generating diversity and adaptation to the environment. The theory of Neural Darwinism proposed initially to apply these principles to the development of the nervous system, with genes being the generator of diversity and selection carried out by a process of maturation. The theory attempted to generalize these mechanisms to physiological processes but it became obsolete because, at this time, it lacked biological incarnation and thus remained on too-abstract a level. It turns on that Neural Darwinism has never been formally applied to the neural processes of decision-making that were not yet formalized at this time.

However, I think that this theory provides a good metaphor here, so I want to pay tribute to its instigators. Following this perspective, the role of the generator of diversity is devolved to the thalamus and the telencephalon and that of the selection engine to the diencephalic and telencephalic loops. The history of the evolution of vertebrates, in which humankind likes to think that they are the ultimate product, could be rewritten as the development of the generator of diversity which allows for the emergence of a very large panel of flexible behaviours.

9
A Hierarchy of Decision-Making

Introduction

So, we will now focus on mammals in order to detail the properties of this telencephalic loop (Fig. 8.2). So far, we have limited our decision-making system to an ultra-simplistic context: two options and binary consequences: reward or not. However, it turns out that in daily life the choices we face are seldom so simple. Therefore it may be useful to examine and classify the different situations in which we have to choose and the modalities involved therein.

A Multi-Option System

Living organisms are seldom faced with choices between two options only; the number is frequently higher. This dimension is also rarely approached experimentally for the sake of simplicity because the number of combinations increases exponentially with the number of options and it thus becomes difficult to collect enough data to obtain robust statistical analysis. But it is generally assumed that the system works with *n* options as with two, and this has been demonstrated both experimentally and theoretically (see Fig. 9.1A).[1]

A Multitask System

Another important property of the system is its ability to make several decisions in parallel. If in the most rudimentary animals, such as lamprey, this

[1] Leblois (2006); Pasquereau et al. (2007); Guthrie et al. (2013)

How the Brain Makes Decisions. Thomas Boraud, Oxford University Press (2020). © Oxford University Press.
DOI: 10.1093/oso/9780198824367.001.0001.

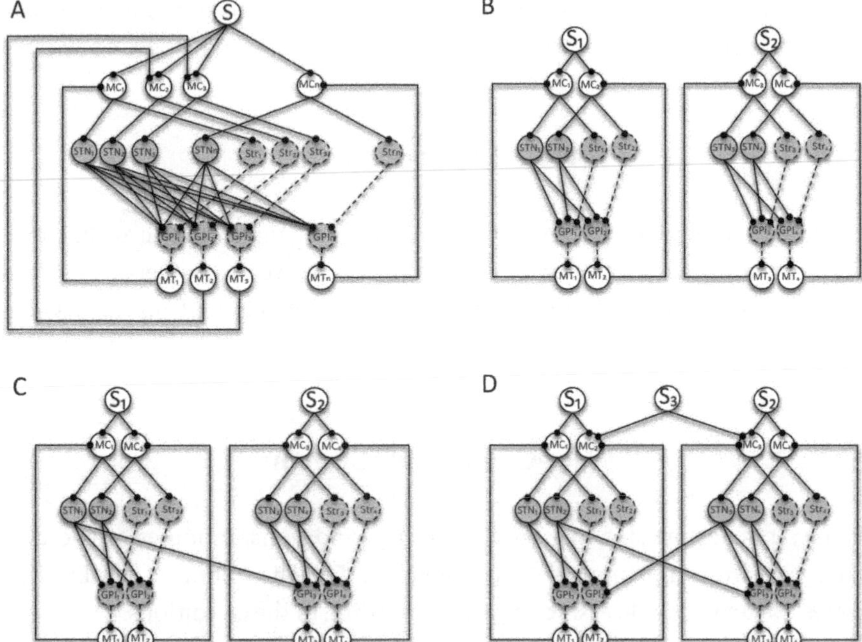

Fig. 9.1 A modular and flexible system. Each possible choice corresponds to a module. (**A**) By increasing the number of modules up to n, we do not modify the dynamic properties of the network. It is still able to activate a single output channel (MC) by inhibiting the others. (**B**) Different assemblies (shown here with only two modules each to simplify the diagram) can operate in parallel without interference. (**C**) By interacting parallel sets, a hierarchy can be installed. In our example, the activation of MC1 will cancel that of MC3. (**D**) Different conditions may cause opposition between modules belonging to different sets, creating de facto new sets. Here stimulus 3 causes a competition between MC2 and MC3. This last example shows that this division into sets is a heuristic device intended to facilitate understanding of the various principles exposed. In mammals, all STN neurons are grouped in the same anatomical structure (the subthalamic nucleus), as well as all the Str neurons (the striatum). For the sake of simplicity, I have not shown here the cortico-cortical connections, but they exist and thus are susceptible to learn also.

property is difficult to highlight, observing the hunting behaviour of a predator is enough to understand that it involves several elementary behaviours in parallel (such as approaching behaviour, scanning for hazards or other predators/competitors, etc.). The system must therefore be able to simultaneously handle several different options without interference. With a modular system like the one we have defined, it is not difficult to design several sets of modules in parallel that can act autonomously (see Fig. 9.1B).

A Hierarchical System

Moreover, it may be interesting for the system to organize itself according to a hierarchical principle: some modules of one set can repress others belonging to another set, in order to prevent two agonistic behaviours from expressing themselves (see Fig. 9.1C).

A Re-Combinable System

Finally, it is conceivable that, under certain conditions, modules of two different sets are competing together (see Fig. 9.1D). The notion of set thus becomes a heuristic artifice, since it varies according to the conditions.

Telencephalic Loop and Ethogram

The system is thus highly versatile and limited only by the number of neurons involved in each elementary behaviour. To examine this question, one can try to compare the number of neurons in the output structure of the basal ganglia: the GPi, which is an anatomical funnel, with the number of elementary behaviours of each species. These data are patchy and difficult to find in the literature, but can be estimated for a few species. In the mouse, this nucleus has a little less than 3,000 neurons; in the rat, this number is about 6,000 (6.10^3); in the macaque, it is above 100,000 (10^5), and in humans, it is close to 700,000 neurons (7.10^5).[2] Concerning the ethograms, the results are even more questionable, but do give an estimate. The mouse has about 13 elementary behaviours; the rat 20; the macaque 130. For humankind, I have not been able to obtain a quantification and it seems that the specialists in human behaviour are reluctant to risk it.[3] Using these values, we can observe that the ratio of the

[2] Extrapolated from Hardman et al. (2002); Herculano-Houzel et al. 2006; Herculano-Houzel et al. 2007; Herculano-Houzel (2009).

[3] Boris Cyrulnik proposed between 100–200, but he carefully stated that this number is hard to obtain and probably under-estimated.

number of elementary behaviours compared to the number of GPi neurons follows a logarithmic law in the other three species (0.005, 0.003, and 0.0004 respectively). This seems logical: what an ethologist defines as elementary behaviour corresponds to a set of micro-behaviours whose number increases as the species becomes more complex. In other words, it takes 200 GPi neurons to subtend an elementary behaviour in a mouse, 300 in a rat, and a little more than 2,300 in the macaque, which, even taking into account my previous remark, allows a margin for some redundancy that is a constant of the nervous system.

If we follow this law, it gives a figure of 150 elementary behaviours for the human species. I have no idea if this figure has any value and I provide it here for informational purposes only.[4]

The Geography of Decision-Making

Let us consider now the topology of these different territories and the major functions with which they are associated. Since the pioneering work of David Ferrier in the early twentieth century, together with the insights of electrophysiology and more recently imaging, we have an increasingly precise understanding of the functional organization of the brain. However, we must be careful not to fall into neo-phrenology, associating a function with a specific brain area, and keep in mind that with regard to decision-making processes (i.e. all behaviour!) it will be necessary to associate cortical areas and territories of the basal ganglia and the thalamus.

Between 1986 and 1990, following the conjoint work of several multidisciplinary teams,[5] a map of the network was broadly defined. Despite some rearrangement, it still remains valid. The network is segregated into five major loops: motor, oculomotor, prefrontal, orbitofrontal, and cingulate (see Fig. 9.2). The first two circuits deal with the learning and decision-making processes of the motor domain. The prefrontal and frontal circuits are involved in cognitive processes. Finally, the cingulate circuit is involved in episodic memory, regulation of emotions (pleasure, fear, aggression, etc.) and modulation of mood.[6] Therefore, we can already see a certain hierarchical order, underpinned by

[4] But this number is compatible with the one advanced by Cyrulnik (see note 3).

[5] Albin et al. (1989); Alexander and Crutcher (1990); DeLong (1990); Albin et al. (1995).

[6] 'In psychology, a mood is an emotional state. In contrast to emotions, feelings, or affects, moods are less specific, less intense, and less likely to be provoked or instantiated by a particular stimulus or event. Moods are typically described as having either a positive or negative valence.' (Wikipedia).

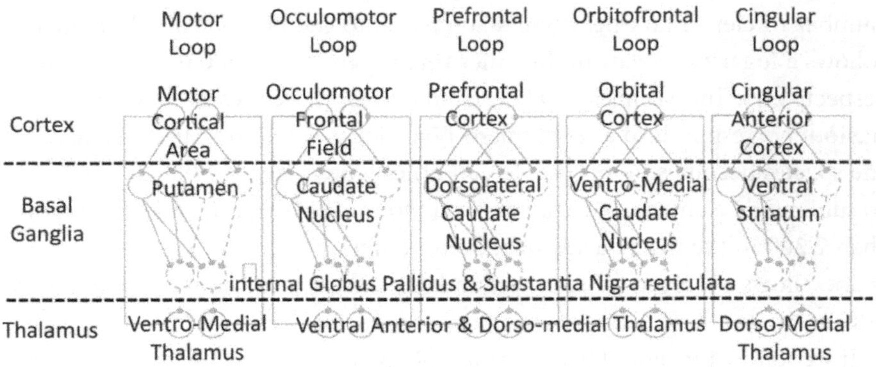

Fig. 9.2 The telencephalic loop is organized in parallel circuits that manage different functions. Each loop is identified according to the cortical areas with which it is associated. We note that these networks are related to different territories of the striatum whose names are provided for comprehensiveness (putamen, dorsolateral and ventromedial caudate nucleus, ventral striatum etc.). Each loop replicates the modular anatomy of the network. Only two modules are shown for each circuit, but there could be many more (potentially 140,000 per circuit if they were distributed equitably, which is probably not the case). The motor, oculomotor, and cingulate circuits operate in an unconscious mode, whereas the prefrontal and orbitofrontal circuits can function in a conscious mode . . . in conscious beings.

anatomical realities: the mood, emotions, and personal history of the subject (his memory) will condition the cognitive functions that will influence motor behaviours. This hierarchy can be concretized by direct interactions between the different loops (see Fig. 9.1C,D) of which anatomical evidence has already been demonstrated several times.[7]

It should not be forgotten that this system is superimposed on the diencephalic loop without replacing it (see Chapter 6). It therefore continues to play a role in visuo-motor coordination and hearing at the very least, but probably in other processes also.

Conscious or Unconscious Choice

We explained in Chapter 2 that when we want to test decision-making processes experimentally, we try as much as possible to free ourselves from the

[7] Graybiel et al. (1994); Kimura et al. (1996); Haber et al. (2000).

notions of consciousness and unconsciousness. There is, however, no fundamental difference between the architecture of networks involved in conscious and unconscious decisions, but simply a different topology. Unconscious decisions involve motor, oculomotor, and cingulate loops as well as the diencephalic loop.[8] Conscious decisions are taken by the prefrontal and orbitofrontal networks.

It is also worth reminding ourselves that the majority of decisions that vertebrates make are unconscious, even if we focus on humans, the only animal capable of self-expressing the notion of consciousness.[9] As far as humankind is concerned, a large part of the behaviour they present in a typical day is based on choices made by their decision-making system that do not reach their level of consciousness. Consider for example the hand we use to open a door: we all use our dominant hand generally speaking (the right hand for the majority of the population), but we will use the other hand without thinking if the first holds a load or if our position in relation to the door does not lend itself to it. The same goes for picking up a cup: we will tend to use the side where the handle is placed, or we will turn the cup without thinking before picking it up. There are a multitude of other examples where humans choose 'without thinking', that is to say without the choice, or even the need to make a choice, reaching their level of consciousness. This allows humans to continue focusing on other tasks.

Thus vertebrates extend their ethogram during the evolution process, thanks to the complexification of the system which is constructed from identical modules but whose functions are diversified and organized in a hierarchical way. However, the basic principles remain the same, the constraints are identical, as are the limitations. It is therefore within the framework of these constraints that the question of the boundary of rationality must be examined.

[8] It is also highly probable that part of the prefrontal and orbitofrontal network also functions in an unconscious mode, if only for species lacking self-recognition capacity.

[9] There is a rich and fascinating debate about the definition of consciousness and the theory of mind in animals. Part of it consists in determining whether the co-operative behaviours observed in certain species (mainly primates) are really motivated by altruistic feelings. At the same time, specialists have not yet decided whether recognition in a mirror is a necessary and sufficient condition for the presence of self-awareness. For a more comprehensive approach see Tomasello (2004) and de Waal (2006) amongst others.

10
Noise and Rationality

(Life) is a tale. Told by an idiot, full of sound and fury.[1]

Variability and Teleology

All behavioural specialists agree that in response to a given problem, the responses of individuals of the same species are variable. This variability is attributed to uncontrolled parameters. Difference in motivation, difference of character, difference in attention or more subtle biological parameters (difference in the concentration of such and such hormones) would be some of the reasons why the experimenter in cognitive psychology or in behaviour must see large cohorts of individuals and many repetitions of the same test in order to derive statistically reliable data.

These explanations are satisfying with regard to the behaviour of several individuals but are less convincing when they are related to the behaviour of a single individual. Here too, variability is the rule. No behaviour follows absolute law and only tendencies can be revealed with more or less important probabilities of occurrence. Let's consider the example of the two-armed bandit protocols (where subjects are asked to make a choice between two lotteries of different values, see Fig. 1.2): after having reached a substantial level of learning, the subjects continue to choose from time to time the least interesting option. We have seen that the traditional explanation involves a balance between exploration and exploitation behaviour. However, this post-facto justification, if it is satisfactory because it provides a simple and comprehensible explanation, also presents the inconvenience of being intrinsically teleological. Indeed, teleology is a major hidden pitfall of neuroscience and biology in general. It is almost impossible to read a publication in neuroscience which does not explain that a particular molecule or structure serves a particular function. As we have already mentioned, what is conveniently called a function in

[1] Shakespeare (*Macbeth*).

How the Brain Makes Decisions. Thomas Boraud, Oxford University Press (2020). © Oxford University Press.
DOI: 10.1093/oso/9780198824367.001.0001.

biology is an emerging property that has been preserved by the mechanisms of evolution because it provides an advantage to the organisms that have it.[2] This is true of all brain functions, from eating to consciousness. To explain a behaviour by the evolutionary advantage that it can possibly induce is to put the cart before the horse.

Noise and Bifurcation

We have seen (Chapter 4) that noise is a prerequisite for the system to generate a choice and that synaptic noise is considered the main source of noise in the nervous system.

At the network level, these phenomena can be amplified by bifurcation processes, especially in networks that rely on populations of excitatory and inhibitory neurons interconnected randomly.[3] This bifurcation phenomenon belongs to what physics calls chaotic processes. It is intrinsically a deterministic process very sensitive to initial conditions (the best known example of chaotic process is the metaphor of butterfly flight in Brazil that is supposed to trigger a storm in Texas). Associated with stochastic phenomena, bifurcation leads to equilibrium states that can be very far apart.

The diencephalic/telencephalic network associates stochastic processes and dynamics that ensure this ability to bifurcate from one choice to another. This process is random at first, and then as learning progresses, the bifurcation will take the most likely path (the one that has been repeated the most times) and that will require the least energy to reach. But due to the stochastic nature of the network, it may happen from time to time that it takes another path and 'chooses' a less interesting option.

Irrational Animals

Thus, the very basis of the apparent irrationality of behaviour is intrinsic to the properties of the decision-making network. This approach is much more satisfactory than traditional explanations because it relies only on biological mechanisms and thus overcomes teleological justifications. Incidentally, it also provides an alternative explanation to individual and inter-individual

[2] See Chapter 7.
[3] Hansel and Sompolinsky (1992, 1993).

variability in behaviour. The variability of behaviour that results from these processes may provide an evolutionary advantage by allowing individuals of each species to be able to switch from exploitation to exploration behaviour. It also adds an additional reason to the various explanations of variability of behaviours of different individuals that remains, even if one restricts the conditions of an experiment to the maximum.

Vertebrates do not behave in an optimized and standardized mode simply because they cannot do it. They are not able to because in order to be able to choose, they need this association between stochastic and bifurcation processes. In fact, the real surprise is more that the notion of rationality emerged from the brain of a big ape. Why did humans invent this concept and how do they manage to use it (theoretically at least)?

PART III
IS RATIONALITY RATIONAL?

11
Reason Under Scrutiny

(Science) is one of the many forms of thought that have been developed by man, and not necessarily the best.[1]

Rationalism and Society

In *Farewell to Reason*, Feyerabend wrote that the rationality of our societies is a myth. He claims that there is always a nucleus of approximation in scientific theories and that the ambition of science[2] to pretend to a universal cosmogony is a dogmatism. In other words, science is only one method amongst others (such as magic, religion, etc.) to explain the world and should not arrogate for itself the right to be the only possible way of thinking, because in doing so, it falls into the same pitfalls as the exclusive religions.[3] This approach, borrowed from libertarianism, is generally rejected by most scientists. But this anathema, apart from the fact that it gives reason to Feyerabend on the dogmatism of science, is based on a misreading. The philosopher does not reject science and religion back to back. According to him, science carries intrinsically an impulse of progress that is absent from religions. Even if science does not always reach its goal, the drive of scientific knowledge is to contribute towards improving human lifespan and quality of life. What Feyerabend is criticizing is the desire of science for universality which, according to him, is a brake on progress. However, the religions to which our societies are confronted also have strong universalistic tendencies and hardly accept to coexist with science (and even less so to coexist between them). If we have to choose between a society

[1] Paul Feyerabend, *Farewell to Reason* (1987). This Austrian philosopher (1924–1994) was inspired by Wittgenstein and Popper. He developed his own philosophy of science based on scepticism about the existence of universal methodological rules.

[2] Here I use the world as a generic word to design every knowledge that is claiming to be based on rationality.

[3] Religions that do not accept any other mode of explanation for the world such as Abrahamic religions (Judaism, Christianity, Islam). Conversely, Asiatic religions (Buddhism, Taoism, Shintoism, etc ...) tolerate each other to the extent that Westerners do not generally grant them the status of religion, but rather that of philosophy. Would philosophy be wiser than religion?

How the Brain Makes Decisions. Thomas Boraud, Oxford University Press (2020). © Oxford University Press.
DOI: 10.1093/oso/9780198824367.001.0001.

governed by science only, with the scientific tendencies that implies, and a society governed by religious dogma, I think that all the examples offered by history and/or recent events demonstrate that the first solution remains by far the best.

It is worth noting that this critical approach to epistemology is contemporary with the demonstration of the limits of human rationality[4] by experimental psychologists[5] and economists.[6] The question is therefore twofold: i) to understand the origins of rationality (even limited) and ii) why it became the dominant mode of thinking in our civilizations. The biologist's answer to the second question is that it provides an evolutionary asset. A civilization that constantly evolves its irrigation system by developing aqueducts, dams, and pumping systems is more likely to flourish than another that depends on rain-making ritual.[7] And we will not dwell on the military, but many historians have shown the preponderant role that the technological development of weapons and the brutalization of the resulting practice of war has played in both shaping Western civilization and ensuring its current supremacy.[8]

Reason and Representation

Where does this obsession with rationality, which imprints its mark on our daily lives, come from? We will not go back to the history of this concept that we succinctly addressed in Chapter 1, but rather to the neurobiological basis. Let us first recall what we define by reason in the context of the study of decision-making processes. To make a rational decision (to exercise one's reason in the context we are interested in) is to choose the option which will be the most beneficial (or the least harmful) according to the information at our disposal.

For that, one must be able:

- to individualize oneself;[9]
- to deliberate;[10] and
- to anticipate the reaction of other individuals.

[4] See Chapter 1.

[5] Herrnstein (1974); Sutton and Barto (1998).

[6] Simon (1947); Kahneman and Tversky (1979).

[7] I borrow this example from Feyerabend (1979): our confidence in rationality leads us to consider the rainmaking ritual as an absurdity, although the inefficiency of this method has never been scientifically demonstrated.

[8] Hanson (1990); Keegan (1996); Diamond (1997); Hanson (2002).

[9] I.e. to identify oneself as an entity.

[10] I.e. to anticipate the consequences of various possible actions.

We humans are capable of conceiving rationality—that is, the possibility of recognizing optimal behaviour in all circumstances—because we identify ourselves as individuals and anticipate the consequences of our actions (and therefore we are aware of our responsibilities) and because we anticipate the reaction of others when they are our allies (we can thus coordinate our actions) or when they are our adversaries (we can thus try to deceive them).

These three capabilities did not develop at the same time during the evolutionary process but stem from a fourth ability, without which they cannot express themselves: the capacity to construct a mental representation of the context. Without this mental representation, there is no possibility of individualizing oneself or anticipating the consequences of our actions in the context of which we execute them.[11]

[11] Here the context indicates both the material environment (place, objects) and other individuals potentially involved (allies and adversaries).

12

Mental Representation

Our life is what our thoughts make it.[1]

The Concept of the Cognitive Map

In 1948, Tolman[2] postulated that spatial learning requires a representation of the environment in which a subject evolves. For example, a rat is able to locate a place that is not directly noticeable by using all the cues available in his environment, regardless of his starting point.[3] Since the animal cannot use a specific cue associated with the goal or reproduce a stereotyped trajectory, it must have a spatial representation that encodes the structure of the environment.[4] This concept has been popularized under the term 'cognitive map', defined as allocentric (independent of the position of the animal) representations of the environment. These maps would retain information about the spatial relationships between different places, which supposes the existence of a coordinate system, or referential.

This hypothesis took time to be accepted. It was the result of a slow maturation and many confrontations between 'behaviourists', who considered the organism as a machine to establish stimulus-response relations, and 'cognitivists', who considered that the subject was able to establish a representation of his environment. Finally, the concept of 'cognitive maps' has been widely accepted. It is now commonplace and found at the heart of memory theories.[5]

[1] Marcus Aurelius, *Meditations* (1995, for the edition consulted). The original quote was in Greek, the language of philosophers in this era. Since television and Internet have replaced the humanities, I would like to remind readers that Marcus Aurelius was the last of the 'Five Good Emperors' and a Stoic philosopher. He was probably not suffocated by his son Commodus, as the bad peplum *Gladiator* suggested (but apart from 1963's *Jason and the Argonauts*, are there good peplums?).

[2] Edward Chance Tolman (1886–1959) is an American psychologist who criticized the rigid concept of behaviourism based only on stimulus-response association (Tolman 1948).

[3] Morris et al. (1982).

[4] In spatial navigation, we can use an allocentric framework (based on the environment) or an egocentric framework (center on the individual).

[5] John O'Keefe, May-Britt Mauser, and Edvard Mauser won the 2014 Nobel Prize for Medicine on account of their work on the neural substrate of the cognitive map.

How the Brain Makes Decisions. Thomas Boraud, Oxford University Press (2020). © Oxford University Press.
DOI: 10.1093/oso/9780198824367.001.0001.

Psychologists describe two types of memory: declarative and procedural memory.[6] The first is the ability to tell an episode from one's previous life (for example, what one ate at the last Christmas meal), to recall the words of a poem or a song, to describe the arrangement of a place that one visited several months ago, or kinship with family members. Procedural memory describes the ability to reproduce learned behaviour (for example, riding a bicycle). We equate this second form of memorization with the decision-making and learning processes that we have described so far. To learn a behaviour corresponds to a sequence of successive decisions which is acquired by trial and error and which does not require a special representation of the environment. On the other hand, declarative memory is based on very different processes. Whatever form it takes, it undoubtedly requires the construction of a mental representation. This mental representation is likened to the 'cognitive maps' theorized by Tolman. This is a generalization of the concept that most likely follows the way in which this ability emerged during evolution. The primitive ability to create a mental representation of the environment was then diverted as new capabilities developed, until the appearance of language.

The Role of the Hippocampus

In 1953, at Hartford Hospital in Connecticut, Dr. William Scoville operated on HM,[7] who was suffering from drug-resistant epilepsy. He was testing a new method to suppress epilepsy which involved surgical lesion of the two hippocampi.[8] The hippocampus is a medial telencephalon structure,[9] folded at the base of the brain in humans (and other primates), consisting of five layers of

[6] As is often the case in cognitive science, there is no consensus and several systems of classification for different types of memory are used. We also find in the literature a subdivision between implicit memory (which is more or less equivalent to procedural memory) and explicit memory (which is partly equivalent to declarative memory). This classification is often preferred by behaviourists because the animals they study do not speak, therefore it is hard for them to declare. In order to be exhaustive, there is also working memory, which corresponds to a memorization in the short term which is probably based on different physiological mechanisms. It can be declarative (a phone number to remember before dialing) or procedural. Since memory is not the subject of this book, readers should refer to the following textbooks: Cowan 1988; Baddeley 1993; Tulving 1995; Squire 2004.

[7] Originally these initials protected the identity of Henry Gustave Molaison (1926–2008). His name is now revealed, but in the literature related to memory, he is generally referred to by his codename, 'patient HM'.

[8] This structure is related to epileptic phenomena, but the full lesion is no longer proposed. Today, neurosurgeons operate in two stages: an exploratory phase when several recording electrodes are implanted in the patient's brain in order to determine the location of the epileptogenic area, which is then secondarily injured. Only very severe cases resistant to all known antiepileptic drugs are treated this way nowadays.

[9] See chapter 5.

cells and divided into several regions named the subiculum, Ammon's horn 1, 2, and 3 (generally abbreviated to CA1, CA2, and CA3), and the dentate gyrus. The operation was almost a total success: the patient never suffered from epilepsy again ... However, he went on to become the number one subject of study for understanding the mechanisms of memory because he developed from that day on a permanent and definitive anterograde amnesia.[10] HM was now unable to fix any new memories for more than a few seconds. He kept intact his old memory until 1942 (11 years before the operation), then it gradually deteriorated. Thus, he remembered that the United States went to war in 1941, but he did not remember either the end date or the way in which the war ended. Only his long-term declarative memory was affected: he could still perform procedural learning.

This clinical case has drawn the attention of physiologists to the hippocampus. Its central role in memory processes has since been confirmed in many species, including the rodent, which is the main study model for this structure.[11]

In the seventies, several teams simultaneously showed that neurons in the CA1 region selectively increased their activity according to certain sensory or behavioural parameters.[12] O'Keefe and Dostrovsky demonstrated that some of these neurons fired selectively when the animal was located in a specific location.[13] They called these neurons, each of which corresponded to a different location, 'place cells'. By simultaneously collecting the signal of several place cells, one can reconstruct in real time the path of the animal in its environment.[14] The whole population makes it possible to form a mental representation of the environment in which the rodent evolves and thus contributes to the creation of this cognitive map conceptualized by Tolman.[15] Since then, the existence of place cells has been confirmed in other mammalian species, including bats,[16] macaques,[17] and humans.[18]

[10] HM's case has been extensively studied by Brenda Milner and Suzan Corkin, two neuropsychologists from McGill in Montréal (Milner and Penfield 1955; Scoville and Milner 1957; Penfield and Milner 1958; Milner 1959, 1972; Cohen et al. 1985; Freed et al. 1987; Freed and Corkin 1988; Corkin 2002; Schmolck et al. 2002; O'Kane et al. 2004; Annese et al. 2014). Histological slices of his brain can be examined on the 'Brain Observatory' website available here: https://www.thebrainobservatory.org/ [last accessed 16 May 2020].

[11] For a more comprehensive approach, I recommend *Memory: From Mind to Molecule* (2009), and *The Hippocampus Book* (2007).

[12] Hirano et al. (1970); Vinogradova et al. (1970); Ranck (1973).

[13] O'Keefe and Dostrovsky (1971).

[14] Muller et al. 1996; Bures et al. 1997; Barry and Burgess (2014).

[15] The contribution of O'Keefe to this work gained him the Nobel Prize in 2014 (see note 5).

[16] Yartsev and Ulanovsky (2013); Rubin et al. (2014). The latter was the first to validate the concept in three dimensions.

[17] Hori et al. (2005).

[18] Ekstrom et al. (2003); Miller et al. (2013).

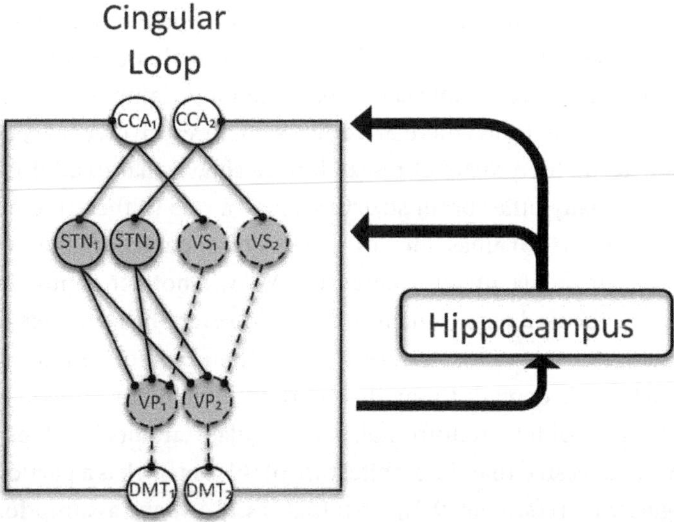

Fig. 12.1 Hippocampus and cingular network. The hippocampus is closely connected to the cingulate loop (one of the subdivisions of the telencephalic loop in mammals) and can interact with it. It is not impossible for it to be a variant of this loop, but this hypothesis remains to be demonstrated. Freely adapted from Retailleau et al. (2012). ACC: anterior cingulate cortex; STN: subthalamic nucleus; VP: ventral pallidum; DM: dorso-medial nucleus of the thalamus. I have not shown here the complexity of thalamic architecture.

In other vertebrates, the medial pallium forms a structure corresponding to a primitive hippocampus. The homology of this structure is strongly suggested by its biochemical and functional similarities with the hippocampus although it does not possess its characteristic shape. Several studies have also demonstrated this functional analogy by highlighting the involvement of the medial pallium in the construction of cognitive maps in birds, reptiles, and fish.[19] Place cells have even been recorded in goldfish![20] It is therefore highly plausible that all vertebrates have the capacity to construct a representation of their environment.

The Memory Networks

Concerning HM, it may be worth mentioning that he only lost the ability to create new mental representations, but that he kept some of those he already

[19] Rodriguez et al. (2002).
[20] Canfield and Mizumori (2004).

possessed. Thus, the hippocampus is involved in the network that allows the learning of these maps, but not in the retention of this information in the longterm (beyond 11 years anyway!). So, if the hippocampus is necessary to create new representations, there are other structures involved, especially in the very longterm. Sixty years of research have shown that in addition to the hippocampus, many other brain structures play a role in these memory processes: different cortical areas, including the ventral part of the basal ganglia, insula, fornix, amygdala, hypothalamus, etc. We will not enter into detail here in order to stay focused on our main subject. However, the processes by which these mental representations are created and then memorized are still very controversial.[21] It is enough to say that among the structures involved, some belong to the prefrontal, orbitofrontal, and cingulate circuits (see Figs. 9.1 and 9.2). We have suggested that the architecture of this network is a particular case of the cingulate loop (see Fig. 9.3),[22] but this is still a vague assumption, based on preliminary data[23] that requires a full experimental demonstration.

[21] Literature is plethoric and theories somehow controversial. Here is a non-exhaustive list of recent reviews: Fouquet et al. (2010); Norman (2010); Rolls (2010); Albouy et al. (2013); McDonald and Hong (2013); Rogerson et al. (2014) ... I didn't even mention neurogenesis; that will bring us further away from our topic, but see for example: Deng et al. 2010; Nogues et al. 2012.

[22] Retailleau et al. (2011); Retailleau and Boraud (2014).

[23] Retailleau et al. (2013); Retailleau and Morris (2018).

13
Mirror, Mirror!

Si le visage est le miroir de l'âme, alors il y a des gens qui ont l'âme bien laide.[1]

Introduction

All vertebrates are thus equipped with the capacity to build a representation of the environment, but we have already seen that this can be far from the case in terms of self-recognition ability. This ability has been demonstrated in only seven species using the mirror test. Six[2] are mammals: the elephant,[3] the killer whale,[4] the bonobo, the chimpanzee, the orangutan[5] and, of course, humans.[6] The seventh animal is the magpie.[7] All of these species have a large brain in common, a large encephalization coefficient, and a cortex (or dorsal pallium) that accounts for more than 50 per cent of brain mass. Brain-imaging studies conducted in humans show that self-recognition strongly involves the hippocampus[8] but especially the prefrontal cortex[9] (or their equivalents), which are two structures more developed in these species than in others. However, it is not certain that self-recognition in a mirror is essential to differentiate oneself from one's fellow creatures.

[1] 'If the face is the mirror of the soul, then some people have a very ugly soul', Gustave Flaubert, *Dictionnaire des idées reçues* (2008, the edition consulted here).

[2] Since I published the French edition, it looks like an eighth species, the rhesus monkey, has passed the test (Chang et al. 2015). It is the first monkey species to do so.

[3] Plotnik et al. (2006).

[4] Delfour and Marten (2001).

[5] Lethmate and Ducker (1973); Povinelli et al. (1993); de Veer et al. (2003) for the three species of great apes.

[6] Postel (1966); Papousek and Papousek (1974).

[7] Prior et al. (2008). The question remains open for other corvids and parrots.

[8] It makes sense because to be capable of self-recognition, one must be able to build a mental representation of self.

[9] Kircher et al. (2001); Sugiura et al. (2005); Uddin et al. (2005).

How the Brain Makes Decisions. Thomas Boraud, Oxford University Press (2020). © Oxford University Press.
DOI: 10.1093/oso/9780198824367.001.0001.

The Mirror Image

In the nineties, in Parma, Giacomo Rizzolatti's team demonstrated the existence of neurons that fire in a similar way when an animal makes a movement, or when the movement is carried out by a third individual. At first these imitation neurons were thought to be isolated in the motor cortex of primates,[10] but they were later identified in other structures[11] and other species[12] and gained the generic nickname of 'mirror neurons'.[13] The discovery of these neurons excited our community and has generated many hypotheses. Some regard these neurons as the basis of empathy,[14] the origin of desire, while others consider them the basis of civilization, nothing less! However, most of these theories, as attractive as they are, have little clear supporting experimental data. But there is at least a very high probability that these neurons are involved in imitation learning processes because they have been found in species that practise this type of learning.[15] This is only a correlation rather than causal evidence, because nobody has yet managed to show that by removing this property, the ability to learn by imitation will also be removed. We must therefore remain cautious about their true involvement in this type of learning, but they do however remain serious candidates. These precautions having been taken, the existence of these neurons challenged the concept that in order to be aware of one's identity it is absolutely essential to be able to differentiate oneself from another. If the mirror neurons excited the neuroscientists so much, it is because the majority of neurons (of the motor cortex in particular) only activate themselves when it is the subject who performs an action. The nervous system of the species endowed with these imitation neurons is thus able to differentiate an action carried out by the individual and another realized by others. Thus, identifying oneself as an individual does not necessarily mean being aware of it. When in doubt, we need to position nearly all mammals and birds (at least songbirds) into the group of animals that can identify themselves as individuals. This solution is compatible with our initial intention to free ourselves as much as possible from the concept of consciousness, a concept which is always

[10] Gallese et al. (1996); Rizzolatti et al. (1996); Rizzolatti et al. (1999).

[11] Fabbri-Destro and Rizzolatti (2008); Caggiano et al. (2009).

[12] Prather et al. (2008).

[13] I am always amazed by the fascination for the mirror among scientists. They could have been called imitation or mimicking neurons, but it seems that the influence of mythology (Narcissus), folktales (Snow White), or psychoanalytic theories imposes this term as soon as the notion of identity is at stake.

[14] Preston and de Waal 2002.

[15] Principally birds and mammals. Learning by imitation is linked to play; see *Animal Play: Evolutionary, Comparative, and Ecological Perspectives* (1998).

problematic in cognitive science, since it makes the notion of the individual independent of self-awareness.

Recognition Processes

According to our approach, individualization and self-recognition are emerging processes of the prefrontal loop which is one of the modules of the telencephalic network we have described (Fig. 9.2). These processes are thus subject to the constraints and limitations of the network. We can infer, for example, that the 6 to 12 months necessary to acquire self-recognition in a mirror for humans[16] corresponds to the learning time of the neuronal populations involved. We have all experienced situations where one wonders 'who is this person who comes in front of me?' in public places with wall mirrors, before realizing that it was actually ourselves. It is very likely that these litigious cases correspond to situations associated with ambiguous information, where the noise switches the system from one state to another and transiently produces a wrong decision.[17]

[16] Wallon (1934).

[17] It is probably worth remembering that we consider that any process of discrimination between several options is a decision. To decide that the image that a mirror sends me is mine rather than that of another is thus an unconscious decision.

14
Anticipation and Utility

A man's worth is no greater than his ambitions.[1]

Introduction

In the previous chapter, I assumed that the processes that make it possible for species to construct mental representations and bring about individualization are based on processes similar to those that make it possible to decide. But what about those processes that allow us to anticipate?

Two processes interact: first of all we need to introduce the concept of delay and therefore temporality, and then we need to introduce a value system.

Time Is Money

Temporality is a complex topic that requires a full textbook to do it justice. Here therefore, we will leave aside the question of the internal clock: how does the brain take into account the passing of time? How many internal clocks are there? What structures are involved? These questions go far beyond the scope of this essay.[2] We will focus instead on anticipation and projection into the future that do not necessarily require taking into account the clock problem.

[1] Marcus Aurelius, *Meditations*.

[2] To my knowledge there is no comprehensive work on this subject (the closest is maybe Buser and Debru 2011). There are several internal clocks, more or less coupled, that are controlled by the neurohormonal system (and we do not even mention here the 'genetic' clock that controls the lifespan of an individual and aging). One of the best known is the circadian clock that controls the sleep-wake cycle that already exists in insects. In vertebrates it is generated by a network involving the hypothalamus and the pineal gland (Harmer et al. 2001; Koike et al. 2012; Woller and Gonze 2013). For shorter time scales (which allow us to estimate time in hours, minutes, seconds, or smaller fractions), the mechanisms are not well known (Buhusi and Meck 2005), but it is likely that the cerebellum as well as the cortex and basal ganglia (hence the telencephalic loop) play an important role (Rao et al. 1997; Harrington et al. 1998a; Harrington et al. 1998b; Bueti et al. 2008). It is assumed that the system relies on several oscillators distributed in several structures that synchronize ad hoc in case of necessity without the underlying mechanisms and the exact nature of these oscillators being well determined (Gupta 2014).

How the Brain Makes Decisions. Thomas Boraud, Oxford University Press (2020). © Oxford University Press.
DOI: 10.1093/oso/9780198824367.001.0001.

Indeed, if many consider that in order to anticipate it is necessary to keep a representation of time, alternative theories postulate that we need nothing more than a decreasing memory system based on the same mechanisms as those of habituation.[3] It is the decrease in the activity of neuronal populations that would manage the notion of the passage of time between two successive events. This idea, which remains to be demonstrated, is interesting however, because it comes close to a property of the process of evaluating the consequences of our actions, which we call temporal devaluation or temporal decay. This concept describes how the value of a reward evolves with the time that separates one from getting it.[4]

When Rats Anticipate the Future

It is thus accepted that the nervous system knows how to manage time (in the form of a clock or in the form of a decreasing function). But is it able to generate anticipatory representations of the future? Since the early 1950s, experimental psychologists have observed that when a rat is involved in an experimental task involving choices, it moves its head alternately in the direction of the various possible options.[5] They called this behaviour 'vicarious trial and error' because they postulated that it corresponded to behavioural evidence of the cognitive processes of anticipatory deliberation (comparison of the different possible options available). Among the arguments in favour of this hypothesis, one of the most convincing was that the frequency of head movements decreases as learning progresses, and then disappears when the performance of the animal is optimal.[6] Moreover, all processes (lesions, administration of drugs, etc.) that interfere with learning, also interfere with these processes.[7]

Due to a lack of evidence, this concept was forgotten until electrophysiology brought it back into consideration. During these episodes of vicarious trial and error, the place cells of the hippocampus and the orbitofrontal cortex were alternately activated as if the animal had made the different trajectories successively several times.[8] The rat's brain was therefore able to build the mental

[3] The process of gradually decreasing the intensity of a response to the repeated or prolonged presentation of the stimulus that triggered it.

[4] A good example of this is that if I ask you if you would prefer to receive 100 pounds today or 120 pounds in six months, most of you would probably choose the first option, even though the inflation rate of recent times has never reached the staggering figure of 20 per cent per year (even with Brexit!).

[5] Taylor and Reichlin 1951; Muenzinger 1956).

[6] Goss and Wischner (1956); Hu and Amsel (1995); Schmidt et al. (2013).

[7] Blumenthal et al. (2011); Retailleau et al. (2013); Amemiya et al. (2014).

[8] Papale et al. (2012); Steiner and Redish (2012).

representation of the path it had to perform for each option. This demonstration has not yet been replicated in other species, but there is no reason to believe that it is different in other mammals or even in other vertebrates.

The structures involved are the same as those that create and maintain mental representations. It is highly likely that the orbitofrontal circuit (see Fig. 9.2) plays a role, even if the scientific evidence for this still needs to be obtained. The processes involved in the selection of an option by the nervous system are based on processes of competition within the telencephalic loop.

Everything Has a Price

Anticipating is one thing, but economists have taught us that in order to be able to choose, one must attribute utility to different options.[9] This utility is subjective and only reflects the subject's preference for an option, but rationality can only be defined if the different options are evaluated according to preference. The eighties played a seminal role for the introduction of this question in the field of neuroscience. It started with Bill Newsome and Antony Movshon, who demonstrated that the activity of neurons in the middle temporal visual area (MT) of the cortex can be correlated with the decisions made by an animal.[10]

Simultaneously, Wolfram Schultz showed that the dopaminergic neurons of the Substantia Nigra pars compacta and the Ventral Tegmental Area play a central role in stimulus-response association processes.[11] But he, and other teams, continued to dissect the properties of the responses of dopaminergic neurons during learning and decision-making processes. They modified their protocol by manipulating the contingency rules (see Fig. 14.1).[12] The different stimuli presented on the screen no longer predicted the administration of a reward a few seconds later, but they were associated with probability. In economic terms, this varied the expected value ($\bar{E}$) of the reward. By recording dopaminergic neurons, as they had done previously, Schultz and his colleagues

[9] See Chapter 1 (Bernoulli 1738; Smith 1778; Samuelson 1938; Houthakker 1950). The neuroscience literature, which is often less sharp on economic concepts, often confounds value, expected value, and utility. I am not sure that the nervous system makes the difference, anyway. Let's remind ourselves that utility is the subjective preference I give to several options (for example, I personally prefer Islay's Scotch to other 'single malt', and 'single malt' to 'blended' whiskies, so I attribute a higher utility to the first than to the second and to the second than to third); the expected value is utility (or value) times the probability of obtaining the option (see Fig. 1.1 in Chapter 1).

[10] See Fig. 3 in Chapter 2; see also Newsome et al. 1989.

[11] See Fig. 6.1 in Chapter 6; see also Schultz 1998b).

[12] For the introduction of this concept, see chapter 1. Let's briefly remind that contingency designates the probability that associates a conditional stimulus with an unconditional one (here a reward).

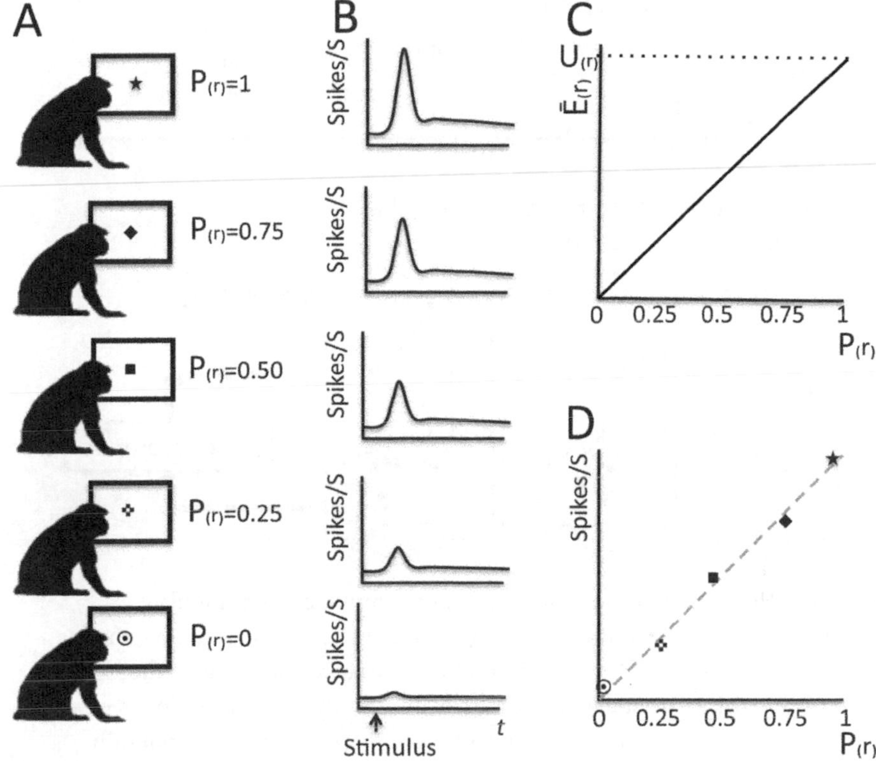

Fig. 14.1 Dopaminergic neurons encode the expected value of reward. This task is very similar to that shown in Fig. 6.1. (**A**) Animals have been trained to follow the appearance of cues on a screen. Different cues predict the administration of a reward (a few drops of fruit juice) with different probabilities (from 0 to 1). (**B, C, and D**) The amplitude of the response of dopaminergic neurons to the presentation of the cues (**B** and **C**) is proportional to its expectation (**C**). From Fiorillo et al. (2003).

showed that the response of dopaminergic neurons to the presentation of visual stimuli varied linearly according to the expectation of the rewards associated with these symbols.

Dopaminergic neurons project significantly onto the striatum, suggesting that this key structure of the telencephalic loop should encode the same information.[13] Subsequently, using 'two-armed bandit' paradigms, other teams have shown that dopaminergic and telencephalic neurons also encode utility during

[13] Apicella et al. (1992); Apicella et al. (1998).

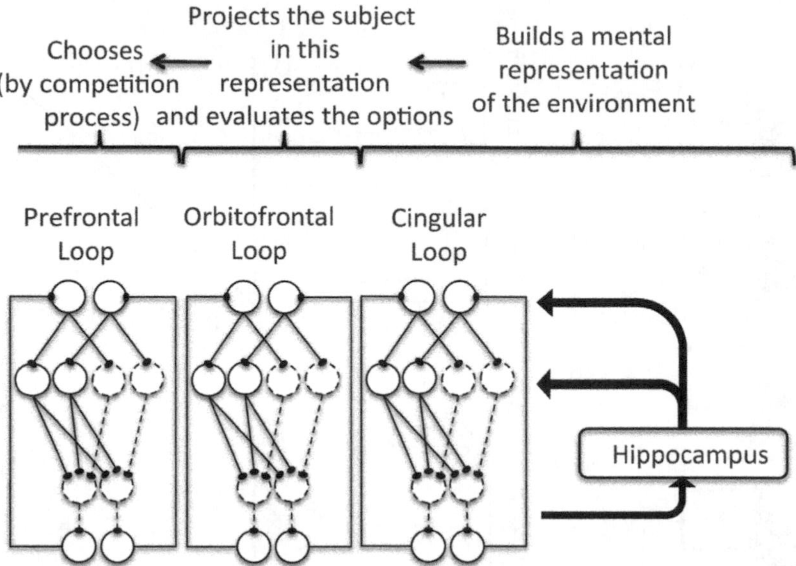

Fig. 14.2 Networks of rationality. The hippocampus and the cingulate loop elaborate a mental representation (cognitive map) of the situation, the orbitofrontal loop projects the subject into the context and evaluates the options, and the prefrontal loop chooses. Naturally, this representation is very symbolic: the boundaries between the different loops are fuzzy and not fully segregated.

decision-making processes.[14] By dissociating the action to be performed from utility, it has been shown both in primates and in humans that there is indeed competition between populations that code for each of the proposed options, and that it is the population that 'wins' this competition that decides the chosen action.[15] Thus, by recording the response of GPi neurons, the main output of the basal ganglia, it is possible to predict the choice made by the subject, even when he chooses the least interesting option.[16]

Since then, many studies have shown that utility[17] is encoded in the orbitofrontal loop,[18] the prefrontal loop,[19] the cingulate loop,[20] and the amygdala.[21]

[14] Samejima et al. (2005); Morris et al. (2006).
[15] Pasquereau et al. (2007); Palminteri et al. (2009).
[16] Garenne et al. (2011).
[17] Or expected value ... neurons 'dont care'.
[18] Gallagher et al. (1999); Kobayashi et al. (2010); Sescousse et al. (2010); Rudebeck et al. (2013).
[19] Rich and Wallis (2013); Vassena et al. (2014).
[20] Vassena et al. (2014).
[21] Rich and Wallis (2013); Rudebeck et al. (2013).

These studies have confirmed the distributed nature of the process between different networks of the telencephalic loop.[22]

Mise en abîme

The previous three chapters have demonstrated that individualization and anticipation of the consequences of own actions, the processes underlying the concept of rationality when applied to oneself, are supported by one or more networks of the telencephalic loop. They should operate on principles similar to decision-making processes, of which they each ultimately represent a particular case. We have discussed in Chapter 9 the possibility of a hierarchy in the functioning of these processes. When we address the problem of rationality we can organize it in the manner of a 'mise en abîme': the limbic loop builds a representation of the environment in which the orbitofrontal loop projects the subject and evaluates the possible options, while the prefrontal loop decides which option to choose (see Fig. 14.2). Each of these loops is subject to the same constraints and is likely to bifurcate occasionally to less 'rational' options because of the stochastic processes involved:[23] to choose the wrong representation (it is not me in the mirror) or the wrong option (the one whose utility is the weakest). If he can talk, the subject will just have to say: 'I do not know what went through my head!'

[22] Samejima and Doya (2007); Guthrie et al. (2013).
[23] See Chapter 10.

15

The Grandmaster and the Playmates

Guess a number from zero to 100, with the goal of making your guess as close as possible to two-thirds of the average guess of all those participating in the contest.[1]

Introduction

Rationality is not limited to the ability to evaluate the consequences of one's actions alone, but also to anticipate those of others. Compared with previous capabilities addressed in this text, the number of species gifted with this ability is drastically reduced. Theory of mind[2] is an almost exclusive characteristic of *homo sapiens*. Chimpanzees are not far off:[3] these animals understand intentions and are able to evaluate the perceptions of others, but they lack the ability to understand false beliefs (where will Maxi search for the chocolate?).

The Beauty Contest

In the thirties, John Maynard Keynes[4] found that across all financial markets, stock prices depended on the perception of market participants rather than their intrinsic value. He concluded that the best strategy for an investor was to guess what others were thinking. To illustrate his reasoning, he chose as an example the beauty contests organized by British newspapers such as the

[1] Challenge proposed in the *Financial Times* in 1997 by Richard Thaler (Nobel Memorial Prize in Economic Sciences in 2017). To be fair, in the French edition my example of the Keynes beauty contest came from a 1983 sample of *Jeux et Stratégie*, the ultimate French geek publication of the era (in fact 'nerd' was more used than 'geek' at this time to designate the population of science-/computer-/comic-oriented young people).

[2] See Chapter 7.

[3] See Chapter 7; see also Call and Tomasello 2008.

[4] British economist who was born in 1883 and died in 1946. The Keynesian macro-economy, of which he was the founder, postulates that the deregulation of financial markets does not lead to an economic optimum. Keynes advocated regulation of the markets. His long-influential vision was rejected by financial liberalism in the eighties. The 2008–2009 crisis generated a renewed interest in his theories.

How the Brain Makes Decisions. Thomas Boraud, Oxford University Press (2020). © Oxford University Press.
DOI: 10.1093/oso/9780198824367.001.0001.

Sunday Times of the Edwardian era: they proposed a panel of one hundred photographs of 'playmates' from which readers (necessarily male, suffragettes had not yet won their case) had to choose the six they considered the most beautiful. The winner of the contest was the one whose choices came closest to the six most chosen pictures. Keynes proposed to standardize his approach by using a mathematical variant of the test, which nevertheless retains its beauty contest name with reference to its origin. In this form, the contest consists of asking a group of subjects to choose a number between 0 and 100, indicating that the winner will be the one who finds the value closest to two-thirds of the average of the proposed values. There is no single solution because the value depends on the level of reasoning (see below) of the majority of the group tested. On the other hand, there is a Nash equilibrium[5]—that is to say a value for which all the participants win—it is the value zero. This is the solution towards which a group converges if it is made to play repeatedly. But whatever the solution, one interesting facet of the game is to provide a classification of the participants into several levels of reasoning.[6]

Level 0: players choose randomly.
Level 1: players assume that the majority of other players choose randomly, so that the average will be around 50 and the value to reach will be around 33.
Level 2: players make the assumption that the majority of the other players are Level 1 and therefore the value to reach is around 22, etc.[7]

There is no absolute level of reasoning. In order to obtain a winning strategy, one must be able to evaluate the average level of reasoning of the other participants, that is, master theory of mind.

This protocol has recently been adapted for fMRI.[8] The authors showed that the activity of the medial prefrontal cortex[9] was positively correlated with the

[5] John Forbes Nash Junior (1928–2015) was the Nobel Memorial Prize in Economic Sciences winner in 1994. He was one of the founders of game theory. His life is romantically told in Ron Howard's biopic *A Beautiful Mind* (2001).

[6] It seems that this classification was proposed by Rosemarie Nagel for the first time (Nagel 1995).

[7] So? Where do you stand in the game proposed in the introduction? In the original contest, the *Financial Times* got 1,382 contestants. The average guess was 18.9, thus the winning value was 13. This meant that the average behaviour was at the second level of thinking, where the winner had to go up to a third level of thinking to win. Regarding the French version of 1983, the majority of readers who answered the competition had used a fourth level of reasoning and therefore the winners had to use a fifth. Please don't infer from this that French people have a higher average level of reasoning; it is more likely to be a bias due to the fact that the publication was geared toward a population of geeks.

[8] Coricelli and Nagel (2009).

[9] This is the part of the prefrontal cortex located inside the hemispheres in the median sagittal plane.

level of reasoning of the subjects. This confirmed what has long been assumed, that the ability to attribute intentions to (and account for) others is correlated with the development of this structure.

The Brain of the *Shogi* Grandmaster

The Japanese developed their own version of the chess game around the sixteenth century. They called it *shogi*. This game presents with a greater mobility and the possibility of reusing the captured pieces of the opponent in his own camp. It results in a much more open game than the Western version, which makes more use of strategic intuition than memorization of combinations. It should be noted that players at international level insist on the Zen[10] aspects of their practice: the best shot to play comes to them intuitively. This is why a number of Japanese researchers use it to study the neurobiological basis of the strategic decision-making in grandmasters of the game. Their work shows in particular that during the phase that precedes the generation of the movement of a piece, the quality of the chosen strategy[11] was positively correlated with the activation of the lateral dorsal prefrontal cortex and the caudate nucleus, i.e. the part of the striatum that belongs to the same telencephalic loop.[12]

Once again, structures belonging to the telencephalic loop are at the origin of the capacity to anticipate the actions of others and to judge their rationality. The prefrontal cortex is the cortical zone that has the greatest expansion in humans compared to other primates.[13] There is no formal data regarding the expansion of associated subcortical structures, but according to the scale laws used in primates, it seems that the progression is linearly proportional.[14] It is therefore possible to imagine a scenario in which the development of the prefrontal loop has allowed the emergence of the ability to anticipate the behaviour of others and allowed the human ape to master theory of mind. So, because of the constraints of the network, which we have already described, even if humans can become experts in anticipating the thoughts of others through learning, due to the nature of the processes implemented, this is not completely foolproof.

[10] Japanese Zen is a practice that insists on 'unthinking'. The Zen master is supposed to act without thinking. From my Cartesian jingoism, I have long thought it was folklore, but I did begin to wonder if, in the end, it does not rely on training the telencephalic loops without activating consciousness.

[11] Assessed using contests similar to the chess game we can find in Western newspapers: 'the white plays and wins in 3 moves'.

[12] Wan et al. (2011).

[13] Van Essen and Dierker (2007).

[14] Herculano-Houzel (2009, 2012a).

Thus, although rationality is at the core of our concerns in Western culture, our mammalian brain is not armed to exercise it fully. We are able to consider different options, to evaluate the one which is the most rational, but we are not always able to choose it, partly because of the stochastic nature of the functioning of our nervous system. This element of randomness is initially a significant evolutionary advantage since it is the engine from which exploration of various options is carried out, enabling us to make decisions, even in times of uncertainty. However, this ability then goes on to turn against us in our quest for ultimate efficiency.

Finally, the remaining question is: 'Is it rational to want to be rational at all costs?' Is this quest not doomed from the start, since we know that we have limits?

PART IV

DO COMPUTERS DREAM OF ELECTRIC BANANAS?

16

The Machine-Learning Approach of Reinforcement Learning

We are machines, stamped out like bottle caps. It's an illusion that I-I personally-really exist, I'm just representative of a type.[1]

Introduction

Our approach, which combines neurophysiology, computational neuroscience, and evolutionary approaches, has led us to postulate that whatever the context, decision-making processes are generated by structures that share a similar architecture and operate in a homologous way. However, this approach is far from consensual. There is a strong tendency in cognitive neuroscience to organize these processes into several distinct and hierarchical systems.

This particular approach is inspired by machine learning. The initial goal of this branch of artificial intelligence, which appeared in the middle of the twentieth century, was to develop and implement algorithms that allow a machine to learn. Originally, they were computers or more or less autonomous robotic automata. As artificial intelligence has developed and cross-fertilized with neuroscience, it has begun to be used to model the learning and decision-making processes for biological agents, broadening the meaning of the word 'machine'. Theoreticians of this discipline define several categories of learning, but we will cover here only those which are related to reinforcement learning.[2]

[1] Quote from *Dick, Philip K. (1996) [1968]. Do Androids Dream of Electric Sheep?. New York: Ballantine Books. ISBN 0-345-40447-5.* by Philip K. Dick (1968). This classic of new wave science fiction describes a universe where corporations are able to create android creatures similar in every way to humans. This is an opportunity for the author to ask the question about what defines humanity? I have always considered that the title is one of the best a novel can carry. Unfortunately, it has since been renamed *Blade Runner* following the success of the movie adaptation (1982). It's a shame that it has lost in poetry what it has gained in brevity.

[2] See Chapters 2 and 4.

How the Brain Makes Decisions. Thomas Boraud, Oxford University Press (2020). © Oxford University Press.
DOI: 10.1093/oso/9780198824367.001.0001.

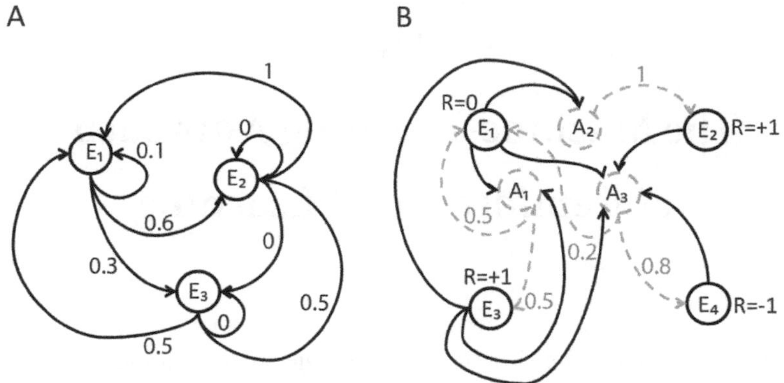

Fig. 16.1 (A) Markov chain. In this example, there are three possible states (E1, E2, and E3) for the system. The Markov chain defines the probabilities of transition from one state to another. Note that the sum of the probabilities of the possible transitions for a given state is always 1 and depends only on the current state. Also note that, in this example, the states are not equiprobable: E1 and E2 are much more likely to occur than E3. **(B) The Markov decision-making process.** In this example, the action (A, in grey) determines the transition probability to the new state. It is thus the sum of the transition probabilities from an action that is equal to 1. Here, the actions A1 and A3 have variable outcomes whereas A2 is deterministic: it automatically leads to the state E2. States are characterized by the reward (R) they provide (here +1, -1, or 0). Note that a given state does not allow all possible actions.

The Markov Chain and Markov Process

To understand how these algorithms work, it is necessary to explain first the Markov chain (see the example in Fig. 16.1A). This is a discrete stochastic process that defines the transition from a state (E) at a given step (t)[3] to the next step (t+1) by a probability function independent of the system history.

Reinforcement learning algorithms formalize the behaviour of an agent in an environment on which it can act according to a Markov decision-making process (see Fig. 16.1B). At each step (t), the interaction between the agent (or subject) and the environment defines a state (E). From this state, the agent must choose an action (A) between several possible options. These actions define a new state at t+1 (which can be the same as the one at t, or a different one). It can produce (or not) a reward value (R). In this context, this term does

[3] We can talk about time or iteration.

not necessarily have a positive connotation because the reward can be positive or negative. The probability of the next state now depends on the action (A) chosen and not on the state (E) at time *t*.[4] In a learning process, the contingency rules between actions (A) and states (E) are unknown at the beginning. It is therefore the role of the algorithm to discover them as quickly as possible, in order to reach an optimum policy.

'Model-Free' Reinforcement Learning Algorithms

In the eighties, Sutton proposed the first real machine-learning algorithm called temporal difference (TD) learning.[5] The principle consists of starting from a situation where all available actions (A1, A2, ... An) from a given state are equiprobable. The function that defines the choice of an action from a state is called policy (π). To evaluate the consequences of this policy, TD learning uses ĒAi(*t*), an estimate of the expected value of the action, between -1 and 1,[6] which is associated with each action Ai(*t*).[7] ĒAi has a value of 0 at the beginning of learning. At each step *t*, the choice of Ai(*t*) will be a function of ĒAi. The algorithm will preferentially choose the action of which ĒAi is the highest. If all utilities are identical, the choice will be random. Once this choice is made, (at *t*+1), the system computes the temporal difference δ(*t*) which corresponds to the difference between Ri(*t*+1), the reward actually obtained, and the expected value ĒAi associated with the chosen action Ai(*t*), all multiplied by a constant. This variable δ(*t*) is also often called the prediction error, which has the merit of being less ambiguous than temporal difference. If δ(*t*) is positive (Ri (*t*+1)>ĒAi(*t*)), then ĒAi(*t*+1) is increased. If δ(*t*) is negative (Ri(*t*+1)<ĒAi(*t*)), then ĒAi(*t*+1) is decreased. If δ(t) is zero (Ri (*t*+1)=ĒAi(*t*)), then ĒAi(*t*+1) is not modified. Thus, as steps proceed, the system will converge to a state where the most interesting actions will be chosen and the others discarded. In the example given in Fig. 14.2, after learning, the system would choose A2 (whose expected value ĒA2=1), when possible, preferentially to A1 (ĒA1=0.5), and avoid A3 (ĒA3=-0.8).

Temporal difference learning and similar algorithms are called 'model-free' learning algorithms. Their shared properties is to track a single parameter: an

[4] But A is not fully independent of E because for some states not all actions are available.

[5] For temporal difference learning, see Sutton and Barto (1998).

[6] It can also be varied between 0 and 1 in which case the starting value will be 0.5.

[7] It may be useful to remind ourselves that the expected value is the mean of the rewards (R) the subject has obtained so far by choosing this action.

estimate of the expected value. The difference between the algorithms relies on the parameters to which the expected values are attributed (the average expectation of an action or that of the states to which the action leads).[8] Amongst them, we can distinguish the greedy algorithms,[9] which automatically select the action associated with the largest estimated expected value, and the stochastic algorithms ('softmax' types), which introduce a random process to allow the system to sometimes choose the lower value options and thus to explore all possibilities. This last class of algorithms is widely used in biology because it is closer to the real behaviour of biological agents that alternate exploration and exploitation behaviour (see Chapter 2).

The Actor-Critic Model

Using this formal description, the actor-critic model that has been proposed represents this approach in symbolic language. It breaks down an agent into two elements: the actor who designates the process that chooses the policy and the critic who evaluates the consequences (see Fig. 16.2).

Model-Based Learning Algorithms

The other family of algorithms that interests us here differs from the previous one through stored information. It is thus the nature of the critic that is different between these two families of algorithms. In model-based algorithms, the whole history of the system is kept in memory. The actor is provided with an anticipatory representation of the cascade of states that he can explore in the following moments, not just at $t+1$. It will therefore be possible to revaluate the estimated expectation of each of its successive actions. If we take the example of Figure 16.1B, a 'model-based' enhancement algorithm will learn to choose A1 rather than A2 because the E2 state to which A2 leads gives no alternative but to choose A3, which has eight out of ten chances of ending up with a negative reward. After learning, the system will eventually result in a stable sequence in which the system will preferentially select A1 to alternate between the states E1

[8] Similar to Q-learning and state–action–reward–state–action (SARSA) learning. For details see Sutton and Barto (1998).
[9] Sometimes called ε-greedy.

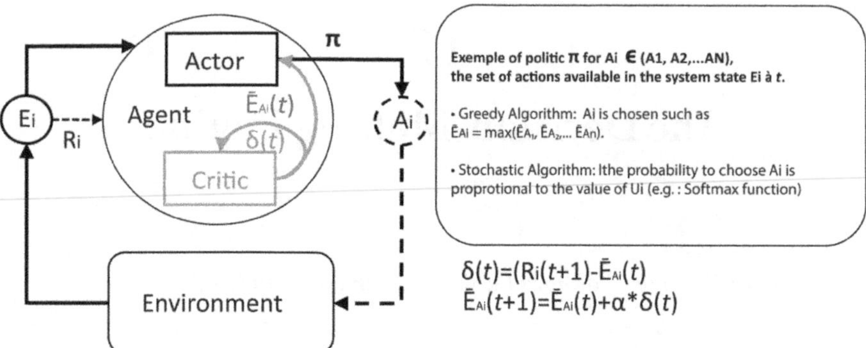

Fig. 16.2 The actor-critic model for a 'model-free' algorithm. The agent is decomposed into two processes: the actor corresponds to the decision-making process: At time *t*, it chooses an action Ai(*t*) from those available according to its policy π (see the box). This action will bring the system (agent-environment) into a new state Ei(*t*+1) associated with a reward Ri(*t*+1). At *t*, the critic provides the expectation ĒAi(*t*) of all the available actions and evaluates at *t*+1, the temporal difference δ(*t*) that will be used to revaluate ĒAi of the chosen action Ai. α is a constant that defines the amplitude of the revaluation of ĒAi.

and E3. The estimated expected value of this sequence will be 0.5 which is the highest value in the longterm.

This example illustrates that model-based learning can lead to better solutions than 'model-free' learning, but it requires many more resources and takes longer to implement.

17
The Decision-Making Engine

A critic is a man who knows the way but can't drive the car.[1]

Dopamine=Prediction Error

Reinforcement learning algorithms, more specifically actor-critic models, are currently very successful in the field of decision-making. They are notably related to properties of dopaminergic neurons not yet addressed in this book.

Indeed, we have seen that dopaminergic neurons respond when the subject receives a reward or when the subject associates a conditional stimulus with the reward (see Chapter 6, Fig. 6.1) and that this response to the stimulus is proportional to the utility function of the reward (see Chapter 14, Fig. 14.1). In fact, dopaminergic neurons behave exactly like a process that computes temporal difference (Fig. 17.1). The amplitude of their response when the reward is administered is proportional to the difference between the expected utility at time (t) and the reward actually obtained at the moment ($t+1$), i.e. the temporal difference. This data was obtained with classical Pavlovian conditioning tasks during which the animal had no action to perform in order to obtain a reward.[2] Later these findings were largely confirmed by other studies using operative tasks such as the two-armed bandit.[3]

To be exhaustive, I must say that the exact nature of the signal produced by dopaminergic neurons is still debated.[4] Some postulate that their activity is correlated to the effort required to perform an action,[5] others to the novelty of a situation or a stimulus.[6] The approach that I have adopted here allows me

[1] Quote from Kenneth Tynan, a British theatrical critic I had never heard of. I have to confess that I found this quote thanks to a search engine.

[2] Fiorillo et al. (2003).

[3] Morris et al. (2004); Morris et al. (2006).

[4] Caplin and Dean (2008); Rutledge et al. (2011).

[5] Salamone and Correa (2012); Nunes et al. (2013).

[6] Zink et al. (2004).

How the Brain Makes Decisions. Thomas Boraud, Oxford University Press (2020). © Oxford University Press.
DOI: 10.1093/oso/9780198824367.001.0001.

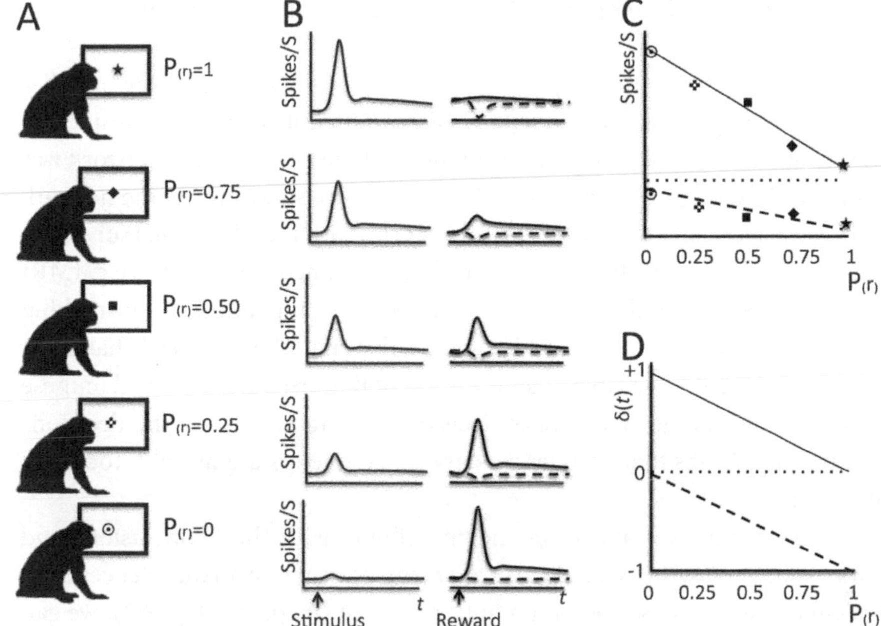

Fig. 17.1 Dopaminergic neurons encode the temporal difference. (**A**) The task is the same as that in Fig. 12.1. (**B, C,** and **D**) The amplitude of the response of dopaminergic neurons to reward (continuous curve) or no-reward (dotted lines) outcome is proportional to the temporal difference $\delta(t)$ (**D**). Note that the slope of the response of dopaminergic neurons is less pronounced for the response to no-reward, than reward outcome responses while the two lines are parallel for theoretical $\delta(t)$. Note also that for the purposes of the experiment, reward was sometimes not administered after a signal that predicted it with certainty. But the ethics is safe because, on the other hand, animals sometimes received a reward after a stimulus that normally announced a certain absence of reward (after Fiorillo et al. 2003).

to free myself from it. Indeed, this debate exists only if one has, consciously or unconsciously, a teleological vision of biology in which functions predefined by a somehow abstract determinism are attributed to networks or molecules. Our approach considers a system in which processes emerge from the system without predefined functions; we do not care if the system we study has only one function or several ... It seems to me more plausible that it has several. So, for us, dopamine can indeed produce a signal similar to a time difference and can also, under certain conditions, play a role in the detection of new stimuli or the quantification of the effort to be produced.

Is the Telencephalic Loop an Actor-Critic System?

Once the observation that dopaminergic neurons transmitted utility[7] and behaved as a temporal difference signal had been identified in the mid-nineties, the analogy between the actor-critic model and the telencephalic network was proposed.[8] This approach attributes to one or more structures of the network the role of actor, and to another the role of critic. Their authors thus substitute two or three equations that can be correlated with neurobiological (e.g. fMRI signals) or behavioural parameters in various learning and decision-making tasks to the complexity of the biological substrate. This approach has been very successful. It has enabled identification of the structures involved in these processes and the noisy nature of decision-making processes. The decision-making algorithms that best describe these parameters are usually stochastic algorithms.

There is, moreover, no major incompatibility with their conclusions and ours. If one applies the symbolism of the actor-critic model to the telencephalic system as we have described it up until now (see Chapter 8, Fig. 8.2), we can propose as a first approximation that the telencephalic network fulfils the role of the actor,[9] while the dopaminergic neurons play the role of interface between the critic and actor. They transmit a utility function at t and the temporal difference $\delta(t)$ at $t+1$. To take this aspect into account, it is enough to slightly modify the initial model and insert a critic module between the reward and the dopaminergic neuron (see Fig. 17.2). This does not modify the dynamic properties of the telencephalic loop. The only modification is that reinforcement learning is no longer done according to a binary mechanism—presence/absence of reward—but according to a scalar quantity that varies between -1 and +1. This signal has two advantages. On the one hand, it directly provides a scalar when anti-Hebbian learning is necessary (if it is negative, then the gain of the activated M-Str synapses is decreased). On the other hand, there is no need to boundary artificially the gain (see Chapter 4), as when $\delta(t)$ is zero, it no longer changes.

However, this analogy has to be considered carefully. First of all, if we are able to describe the dynamic properties of the actor network precisely enough, there is currently no sufficiently accurate anatomo-physiological data to produce an equivalent of the critic network. What we can say is that it must involve

[7] Schultz et al. (1997)

[8] Houk et al. (1995); Doya (2000); Daw et al. (2005); Daw et al. (2006); Schultz (2006); Daw (2007); Samejima and Doya (2007); Humphries et al. (2012); Khamassi and Humphries (2012).

[9] In lower vertebrates the diencephalic loop is substituted for the telencephalic one.

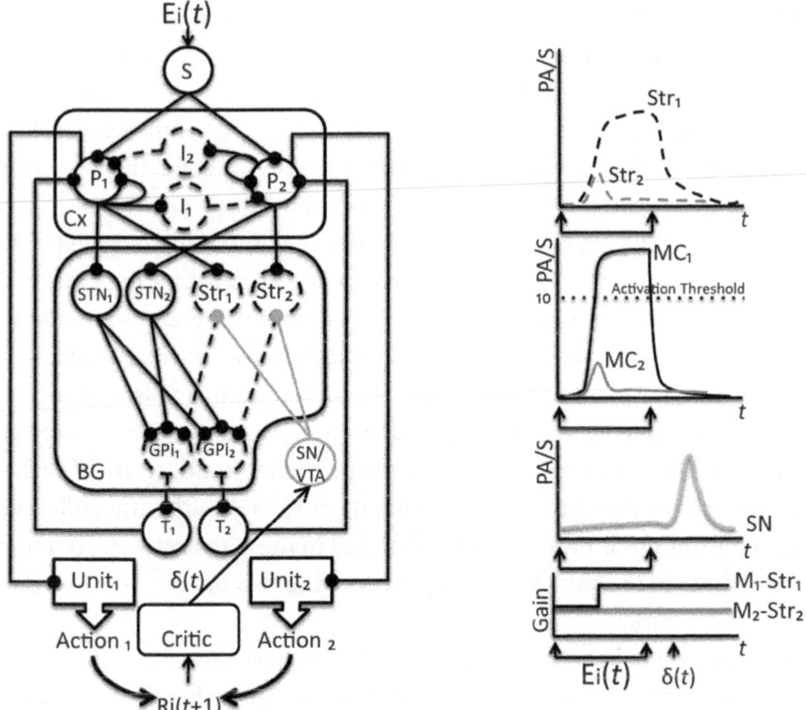

Fig. 17.2 The telencephalic network adapted to the actor-critic model. The architecture of the telencephalic network is not modified as compared to the initial one (Fig. 8.2). It fulfils the role of the actor. It chooses an action in response to a state Ei(t) at time t. It is the architecture of the loop that determines the followed policy. In this case the behaviour of the loop can be fitted with a softmax type algorithm. On the other hand, the dopaminergic neuron (SN) no longer codes directly Ri (t+1), the presence or absence of the reward at t+1, but the temporal error δ(t). This is generated by a critic network embedded between the reward and the dopaminergic neuron. It is therefore δ(t), and no longer the presence or the absence of reward, which will modify the Hebbian learning processes at the cortico-striatal synapses (M-Str).

the dopaminergic neurons of the Substancia Nigra pars compacta and Ventral Tegmental Area and therefore probably the areas connected to them. Among these, we have already presented some: the striatum of course, with which these structures are connected in both directions, but also the ventral part of the globus pallidus. There are also others of which we have not yet spoken, including the amygdala, the lateral habenula, and mesencephalic structures such as the pedunculo-pontine nucleus and the raphe nuclei. The network must probably also involve other structures that are connected to them: notably the orbitofrontal cortex, the anterior cingulate cortex, and the hippocampus. We know that the activity of the three structures is correlated with reward, utility, or temporal difference.[10] Some of these structures are part of the telencephalic network, to which has been attributed the function of the actor, therefore it appears difficult to clearly segregate the two processes.

The nature of the signal propagated by the dopaminergic neurons at the initial step is another pitfall. It is relatively established that dopaminergic neurons behave in a homogeneous way. They cannot therefore provide the utility associated with each available action, but only an average utility of all the possible actions.[11] If one remains stuck on a rigid formalism, this question remains insoluble. But our approach shows that the gain of cortico-striatal synapses (M-Str) is specific and proportional to the utility of each of the actions for which a population of striatal neurons is coded. The difference between the options is thus already embedded in the actor network. It underlines the limits of the complete segregation of the two processes to two fully segregated networks.

On the other hand, the time dimension that we have not taken into account up until now posits a still unsolved problem: the delay between the action performed and the reward provided. If we consider that $\delta(t)$ allows readjustment of the weight of the cortico-striatal synapses,[12] it is necessary to add to the standard RL mechanisms another which allows it to keep a memory of the activated synapses. This is referred to as eligibility trace.[13] It seems that the answer exists in the phenomenon of time-dependent plasticity processes that have been studied for more than ten years in the striatum, but there is still no consensus.[14]

Convergence of Connectionist and Automatic Approaches

The model-based approach has been introduced relatively recently in the field of cognitive neuroscience. It shares many analogies with the concepts of

[10] For review, see Haber and Knutson (2010).

[11] Morris et al. (2006).

[12] It could be inferred that the dopaminergic signal transmitted at the time of the presentation of the stimuli plays this role, but this solution would simply shift the learning process. This artifice also raises another problem which is that of the way the critic learns. It is very likely that the striatum plays a determining role in the evaluation function and as such, it must be able to integrate $\delta(t)$ to revise its utility functions (and thus plays an active role in the critic process also).

[13] Florian (2007); Killeen (2011); Saito et al. (2011); Vassiliades et al. (2011).

[14] Caporale and Dan (2008); Fino and Venance (2011); Feldman (2012).

mental representation, cognitive maps, and deliberation. It has been proposed as a complement to the model-free approach, assuming that the two processes are in competition and underpinned by very different networks.[15] However, starting from a purely automatic approach, Khamassi and Humpries have proposed a theoretical model from which they draw conclusions very close to ours.[16] They posit that: i) the cingular loop (see Fig. 9.2) builds the model of the environment, i.e. the representation of all the stimuli, states, actions, and rewards that define the environment; ii) the orbitofrontal and prefrontal circuit works like a model-based algorithm, which evaluates the utility of each option according to all the information available in order to develop 'directed' behaviours (we would say rational in our context); and iii) the motor circuit works like a 'model-free' algorithm to build 'habits' which are stimulus-response association sequences.

The Limits of the Automatic Approach

It is therefore possible to use reinforcement learning algorithms to study the behaviour of the telencephalic/diencephalic network in the learning and decision-making processes that we have described so far. The advantage of this approach is to be able to model them with very few parameters and a handful of easy-to-code algorithms to replicate these behaviours with virtual or real robots.

This formalism converges with our approach and leads to conclusions that are quite similar to ours concerning the structures involved and the stochastic nature of decision-making. It has the heuristic advantage to clearly explain the function of the networks studied.

But this advantage is also a drawback. On one hand, it induces an underlying teleologism that is antagonistic to the repositioning of the question in an evolutionary perspective. It easily misleads to the identification between a function and a structure of which the neural activity correlates vaguely with an algorithm. This type of reasoning is also at the origin of the parochial quarrels that regularly animate the scientific community because correlations are generally found in different structures as it is expected in a distributed process.

[15] Daw et al. (2006).
[16] Humphries et al. (2012); Khamassi and Humphries (2012).

Moreover, these algorithms are purely descriptive. If they insist, as we do, on the stochastic nature of decision-making processes, they do not explain their origin. Thus, they are able to replicate the limits of our rationality but are unable to explain why. When they are used, one should keep in mind that this is a description, not an explanation, in order not to overshadow the understanding of how function emerges from the process.

PART V

RATIONALITY, FINAL FRONTIER

18
Bias and Heuristics[1]

Introduction

Whether with the connectionist approach that we have adopted, or an artificial intelligence approach, we have converged on the observation that the processes implemented for decision-making do not completely obey the principles of rationality and are subject to a certain degree of randomness. The connectionist approach coupled with an evolutionary dimension provides an intrinsic explanation: we are not rational because the principles of rationality emerge from a structure that has no finality in itself. Stochasticity is a necessity for the system to be able to make choices. Learning processes have emerged from the substrates involved in eating behaviours to improve performance. Ethograms then developed in parallel with the pallium mantle and its complexification, which introduced more regularities and automatisms, the roots that enable the development of skills and habitual behaviour.[2] Finally, the ability to produce mental representations eventually emerged and provided the necessary substrate to anticipate and thus to conceive of rationality.

As we have already stated,[3] the notion of rationality is an avatar of these processes, not necessarily shared by all humanity, but central to Western civilization, of which it is one of the cosmogonic principles. However, even if our civilization claims to be based on purely rational principles,[4] irrationality still permeates. To avoid making myself too many enemies, I will simply give as an

[1] Part of the materials of this chapter has been published in Boraud et al. (2018).

[2] Boraud et al. (2018).

[3] See Chapters 1 and 10.

[4] Let's remember that according to the economic principles that govern us, the markets do not need to be regulated because the economic agent is supposed to behave as a purely rational entity.

How the Brain Makes Decisions. Thomas Boraud, Oxford University Press (2020). © Oxford University Press.
DOI: 10.1093/oso/9780198824367.001.0001.

example the omnipresent horoscopes in newspapers and the success of homeopathy, where the effectiveness of one or the other has never been scientifically proven. It is true that their ineffectiveness has not been scientifically proven either, but no scientist worried about his own reputation would try to do this since the Benveniste affair,[5] thus showing a risk aversion that is not necessarily more rational. Rationality is therefore at worst a myth, at best an approximation.

Heuristics in Judgement

Herbert Simon[6] introduced the notion of heuristics in judgement to define the approximate rational rules upon which individuals rely to make decisions. Tversky and Kahneman transformed this notion of heuristics by highlighting the cognitive biases that influence judgements. The theory that formalizes their work (see Chapter 1, Fig. 1.3) considers some of these factors, including the way in which subjects asymmetrically assess their prospects for loss and gain and risk aversion.

The Quick and the Slow

From his work with Tversky, Kahneman elaborated on the two-systems theory.[7] According to him, human decision-making is the result of a competition between a fast, automatic system (System 1) that is prone to make mistakes and a slower, more demanding but also more reliable system (System 2). Both systems use heuristics, but the second compensates with anticipation. Kahneman himself never identified a neuroanatomical substrate for his theory, but many others have tried to place it in parallel with the theory of triune brain organization:[8] the fast system being associated with the 'reptilian brain', while

[5] Readers over 40 will remember the scandal of the 'memory of water' in the 1980s following the publication of the work of Benveniste who claimed that molecules of water retained an electromagnetic trace of molecules in high dilution, even at infinitesimal concentrations (Coles 1988, 1989; Thomas 2007).

[6] Simon (1955).

[7] Kahneman (2012).

[8] A theory popularized by MacLean (1973) in the sixties that divides the brain into three stages of development; the reptilian brain, the limbic brain, and the neo-mammalian brain. Each stage adds new behavioural features to the ethogram. The reptilian brain corresponds significantly with the diencephalon and the basal ganglia and is responsible for instinctive behaviours (aggression, dominance, territoriality, ritual displays, etc.). The limbic brain is involved in feeding, reproductive and parental behaviours, with the ability to display motivation and emotion. The neo-mammalian brain allows us

the slow system is identified as a product of the 'neo-mammalian cortex'.[9] In fact, our approach is quite the opposite: the slow system would be supported by the older reinforcement learning-dependent cortico-subcortical loop, while the fast system would result from cortical Hebbian associations (see Chapter 8, Fig. 8.3). This implies that shortcuts (heuristics) rely on cortical processes whilst deliberating decisions and actions, which rely on emotional and moral motivation, rather stand on a subcortical substrate. However, the identification is incomplete. We saw earlier (Chapter 12) that the capacity to anticipate is underlied by a network encompassing the prefrontal cortex and the hippocampus. Therefore, System 2 also needs to interact with this network in order to be able to compensate with anticipation. Considering these anatomical constraints, our approach brings a fresh view to the psychology of decision-making and may help to unravel the neural correlates of cognitive bias.

Initial Bias and Beliefs

So far, we have assumed that when an agent is immersed in a new environment, he is genuine and has no history. The utility of the options available to him are unknown and his choice depends only on the noise generated by his decision-making system. But in fact, this is barely the case. Our decisions are very often biased a-priori, their origins multiple. These initial biases may result from a poor mental reconstruction of the situation. This may be having preferences for dimensions that are not relevant to a task. For example, it has been observed in two-armed bandit paradigms that animals have displayed a preference for a cue's colour, or a direction, two dimensions that are not relevant in our tests. They therefore do not choose according to the highest probability of reward.[10] In 'beauty contests', it is not uncommon that when the individual who gave the answer closest to the requested value is asked how she has defined her choice, the answer is: 'it's my lucky number'. So wrong reasoning can bring a good solution. In general, learning processes usually correct these biases, and animals

to perform abstract thinking, planning, and, for the most advanced species, use language. Each level inhibits the lower one. The key to human neuropsychiatric pathology stems from defects in these inhibition processes. Triune brain theory was widely accepted because of its elegant ability to link between structure and function, and its vague similarities with Freud's psychoanalysis theories. Despite being widely refuted by specialists in neural development and physiologists, this theory is still influential in cognitive sciences. For a more comprehensive critique of triune brain theory, see Boraud et al. (2018).

[9] E.g. Crosby (2015).

[10] Laquitaine et al. (2013).

that choose early on the wrong criteria usually correct their mistakes after several dozens of tests.[11]

The Anchoring Effect

Anchoring is the excessive influence of a first impression on judgements. It is one of the important elements of the framing effect underlying prospect theory. It can take different forms. A first example is that the price proposed at the beginning of a negotiation influences the outcome. Another example is the way in which a problem is stated (saving 200 out of 600 people or leaving 400 to die)[12] that modifies choice. A final example I will give is the influence of that first gain in a gambling game that is an important predictive factor in the development of a gambling addiction.[13]

Amongst these three examples of anchoring effects, the last one is the easiest to predict from our model. The initial reward biases the system because the temporal difference δ(t) is very high. This results in a high modification of the gain of the cortico-striatal connections of the modules corresponding to the gaming behaviour in the orbitofrontal network which will therefore favour the selection of this type of behaviour (see Fig. 18.1).

The two other examples are more complex to formalize because they are more abstract in behavioural terms.

Regarding the former, we can nevertheless imagine that in the first case the anchoring phenomenon is explained by providing a mental representation to the cingular network which in turn provides a reference of utility. In the absence of other information, the temporal difference δ(t) is computed with respect to this value, biasing the decisions of the subject accordingly.

For the second example, let's remind ourselves to start with, that if one proposes to choose between saving 200 people out of 600 for certain or having a one in three chance of saving 600 people, the subject prefers the first policy, whereas if the question is formulated 'would you prefer to let 400 people die for certain or to have two chances out of three to see 600 people die', the preference would be rather for the second proposal. This paradox is predicted by prospect theory (the combination of risk aversion and overvaluation of losses). Our approach does not bring much more. We can nevertheless model that the anchor

[11] *Ibid.* 249.
[12] Kahneman and Tversky (1979); see also Chapter 1.
[13] Thaler and Johnson (1990).

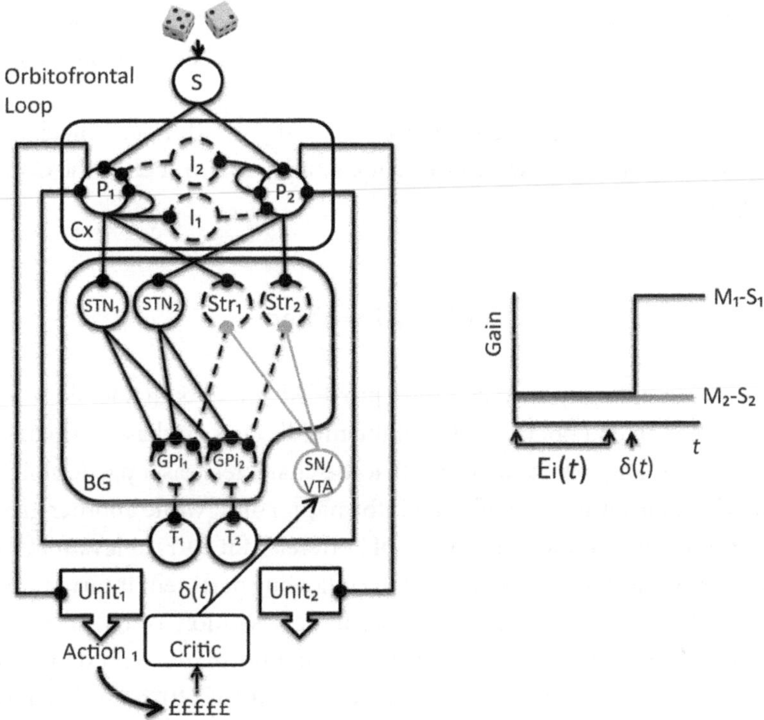

Fig. 18.1 The impact of the first gain. The subject who tries a gambling game for the first time knows that his chance of winning is low. The utility function is therefore almost zero. If, by chance (or by perversity on the part of the game provider), he wins a large sum on his first try, the temporal difference $\delta(t) = R(t + 1) - U(t)$ is much greater than zero and therefore the gain of the cortico-striatal connection associated with the game behaviour is greatly increased. This will result in a reinforced learning behaviour. This element is a significant risk factor for gambling addiction, but it is not the only one. In the majority of subjects, several successive negative temporal differences will be responsible for bringing the player back to reason.

defines the reference against which the temporal difference is computed by the network. Thus, while the subject evaluates the outcome of his choices using anticipation, he will estimate $\delta(t)$ as follows:

- In the first case $\delta(t) = 0$ (he hopes to save 200 people and he saves 200).
- In the second case $\delta(t) < 0$ (he hopes to save 600 but he saves only 200, probably less because of his poor estimation of probabilities).
- In the third case $\delta(t) = 0$ (he expects to see 400 people die and 400 die).

- In the last case $\delta(t) > 0$ (because he expects to see 600 people die, but 'only' 400 die, or even less because of his poor estimation of probabilities).

The three anchoring effects described use slightly different mechanisms, but all involve the way in which the 'critic system' will influence the decision-making process.

The Dilution Effect

A (not truly politically correct) study provided students in sociology with a brief description of a 'social worker of the middle class' and asked them to decide if it was highly probable or not that the character was a paedophile. One group of students was given relevant information only, while another group of students was provided with a mixture of both relevant and irrelevant information.[14] For example, they were offered the following pertinent information: 'He was sexually abused by his father-in-law', or 'he has sadomasochistic fantasies', or 'he has a drinking problem' . . . The irrelevant information could include the following: 'He runs a hardware store', or 'he has an IQ of 110', or 'he lost two fingers from his left hand'.[15]

Subjects who received both types of information felt that the individual was less likely to be a paedophile than subjects who received the relevant information only. According to the authors, irrelevant information would make the individual appear less representative of a paedophile. They called this phenomenon 'the dilution effect'. This effect can be explained quite easily with our own model. We have proposed that mental representations are formed through competition mechanisms identical to those used in decision-making (see Chapters 11 and 12). In other words, our brain 'decides' on the contours of the mental representation that it builds. Consider that each piece of information activates an elementary module in the cingulate circuit of students trying to build a mental representation of this social worker (see Fig. 18.2). If the information provided activates only circuits carrying relevant information, the mental representation will conform more easily to the desired model. On the other hand, the more the information activates irrelevant modules, the weaker the interactions will be, and the more the information that will win

[14] Nisbett et al. (1981).

[15] I leave to the authors of this study the responsibility of the actual relevance of the information provided!

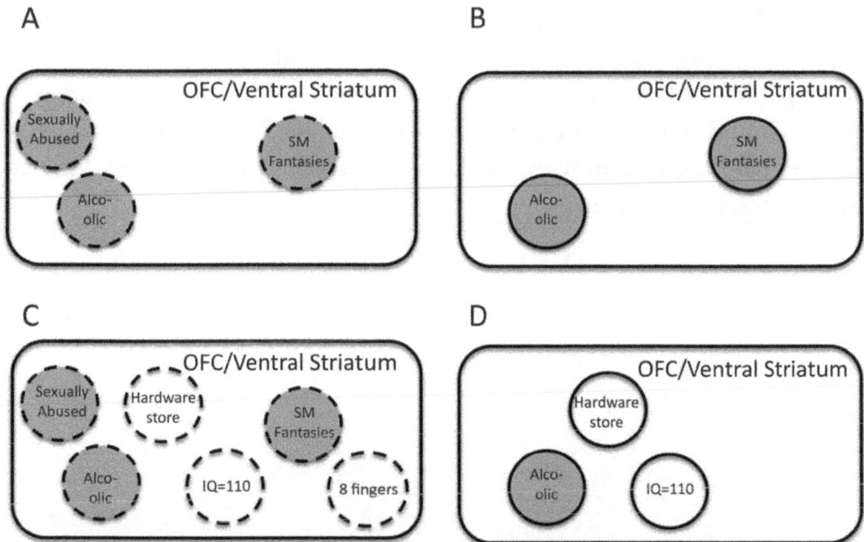

Fig. 18.2 The dilution effect. If only relevant information (in grey) is presented (in black) to the subject (**A**), changes in cortico-striatal gains will favour the creation of congruent mental representations (in grey) in its cingulate network (and associated hippocampus) with the sexual orientation of the individual described (**B**). If irrelevant information is presented jointly (**C**), the probability of congruence of the populations that will be consolidated decreases. The final representation may thus move away (**D**). I will let readers judge the good taste of the examples used by psychologists in this experiment.

the competitive process that governs the creation of this mental construct will move away from the archetype and so the probability of identifying it decreases.

Finally, what is our contribution to the debate? Through these three examples, we have shown that by dissecting the neurobiological substrate of decision-making—a change of state within a neuronal population made possible by the combination of stochastic and chaotic processes—we provide a physiological explanation for the heuristics in judgement that underlie what Dan Ariely calls the irrational predictability of our behaviours.[16]

Economists and psychologists have formalized the existence of these biases, while we have provided an explanation for some. We know that they are written in our nature, so it is not a matter of fighting against them, but rather of

[16] Ariely (2008). I recommend his TED talks, notably: http://www.ted.com/talks/dan_ariely_asks_are_we_in_control_of_our_own_decisions [last accessed 17 May 2020].

living with them. Based on these observations and detailed characterizations provided by studies in behavioural economics, it might be interesting to try to develop more relevant judgmental heuristics than those that come more naturally to mind. The range of applications for such methods is vast: expert systems, economics, education, road safety, medicine, functional rehabilitation, and defence, to name a few.

19

Pathologies of Decision-Making

Never put off till tomorrow what you can do the day after tomorrow just as well.[1]

Introduction

If we are not fully rational, we manage to pretend to be most of the time. Some individuals are distinguished by traits that influence their decision-making: impulsiveness, procrastination, stubbornness, etc. These behaviours are so common that they are not considered pathological. There are, however, cases in which the decision-making system is dysfunctional enough for this irrationality to go beyond socially acceptable norms. This is the field of neurological and psychiatric syndromes of decision-making.

Obsessive Compulsive Disorders

Obsessive compulsive disorders (OCDs) are mental disorders characterized by the repeated appearance of intrusive thoughts—obsessions, anxiety—accompanied by repeated and ritualized behaviours—compulsions—which can have the effect of reducing anxiety. It affects about 2.5 per cent of the population. Obsessions and compulsions are not always associated. The individual suffering from OCD recognizes its irrational character but he cannot repress it and it reduces the time available to him for other activities. The *Diagnostic and Statistical Manual of Mental Disorders* (*DSM-V*) (the gold standard in the classification of psychiatric disorders) considers that an individual suffers from

[1] This quote is usually attributed to Oscar Wilde. It seems to be an invention of one of his biographers while the original quotation is by Mark Twain who apocryphally attributes it to Benjamin Franklin. It is amazing how much useless information can be found on the Internet when you have procrastination tendencies ... well, I'll go back to my book now.

How the Brain Makes Decisions. Thomas Boraud, Oxford University Press (2020). © Oxford University Press.
DOI: 10.1093/oso/9780198824367.001.0001.

OCD if compulsive activities consume him for more than one hour per day. This is a way of recognizing that we all suffer more or less from obsessions and compulsive behaviours and that it is therefore only a question of the threshold of tolerance.

Physiopathological studies on human subjects or animal models of the disease show hyperactivity in the orbitofrontal circuit (see Chapter 9, Fig. 9.2) in correlation with obsessions or verification behaviours. It has been shown in the orbitofrontal cortex, the ventral part of the caudate nucleus, the ventral part of the subthalamic nucleus, and ventral anterior and dorsomedial thalamus.[2] It is postulated that this is a hyper excitability of the network that switches to a state of selection by a defect in the stabilization system. Our model makes it possible to explain it from the study of the dynamic states of the network as a function of the overall synaptic coupling strength of the positive feedback pathway (G+) and the lateral inhibition pathway (G-). This hyper sensitivity causes an increase in the gain of the direct path (G+). This results in a transfer of the system into a regime where the activation of certain modules of the orbitofrontal circuit is spontaneous (see Fig. 19.1). That's what generates obsessive ideas. Compulsive behaviours would aim to stimulate other cortical modules to switch the circuit to another state. This explanation is hypothetical but provides an interesting track.

Tourette's Syndrome

Tourette's Syndrome is a pathology similar to OCD, with which it shares a certain comorbidity (which could be up to 80 per cent).[3] It affects 1 per cent of adults and 0.4–3.8 per cent of children under 18.[4] It is characterized by behavioural twitches—eyelid spasms, head movements, barking, grimaces etc.—and language stereotypes: coprolalia (compulsion to pronounce profanities), echolalia (repetitions of the sentences of others), or palilalia (repetition of one's own sentences). The pathology is also characterized by functional anomalies that affect the motor circuit of the telencephalic loop.[5] Less well characterized than OCD, it is more difficult to have a clear vision of the pathophysiological process implemented. However, due to its high comorbidity with OCD, it may be suggested that these are similar mechanisms (see Fig. 19.1) but that they affect the

[2] Guehl et al. (2008); Rotge et al. (2010); Welter et al. (2011); Rotge et al. (2012); Burbaud et al. (2013).
[3] Cavanna et al. (2009).
[4] Robertson (2011).
[5] Ganos et al. (2013).

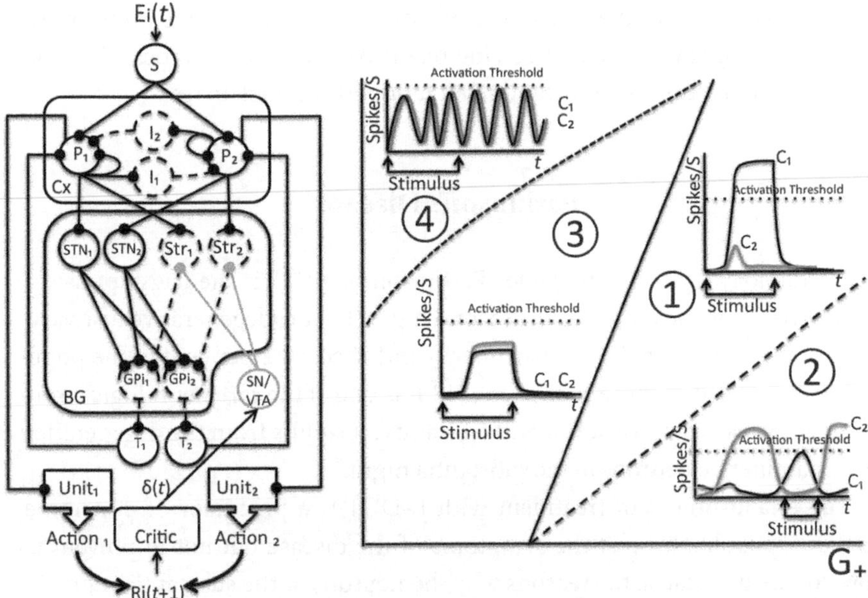

Fig. 19.1 Physiopathology of the telencephalic loop. The dynamic regimes (modes of operation) of the telencephalic loop represented as a phase diagram of a function of the gains of the positive feedback path (G+, on the x axis) and that of the gains of the signal path, inhibition (G-, y axis). Under physiological conditions (1), the system is able to choose by specifically activating a population of cortical neurons (C1 in the example). In the case of OCD or Tourette's syndrome (2), C2 spontaneously activates without stimulus triggering stereotypical behaviour (OCD or tics). In the first case, the pathology reaches the orbitofrontal circuit, in the second, the motor circuit. A stimulus (compulsion in the case of OCD, focusing on tics) can stop unwanted activations by causing the activation of a module in competition, but the very unstable system can switch again when stopped. In the case of Parkinson's disease (3 and 4), the telencephalic loop is no longer able to choose between C1 and C2 in response to a stimulus. Note that there are two 'parkinsonian' conditions including one (4) in which the system oscillates. This accounts for oscillations that are often (but not always) found when the electrophysiological activity of patients or animal models of the disease are recorded (Leblois, Boraud et al. 2006).

The oscillation problem goes beyond the scope of this book, for more details readers can refer to Brown (2003); Leblois et al. (2006); Dejean et al. (2008); Degos et al. (2009); Dejean et al. (2012); Syed et al. (2012).

motor circuit. Due to the hyperexcitability of the network, some motor modules activate spontaneously, triggering repetitive motor stereotypes. Here too, this hypothesis requires verification, but it provides a track to test.

Parkinson's Disease

The pathology described by James Parkinson in 1817[6] is the flagship disease of the telencephalic loop. It is the second highest neurodegenerative disease in terms of frequency (behind Alzheimer's) and affects 0.2 per cent of the population (1 per cent of those aged over 65).[7] It is one of the rare neurological syndromes whose origin we know with certainty: it results from the degeneration of dopaminergic neurons in the substantia nigra.[8]

The establishment of treatment with L-DOPA, a precursor of dopamine, makes it possible to treat the symptoms of the disease but not to prevent its development, because the reasons why the neurons of the substantia nigra die faster than others are not yet known. These are probably multifactorial mechanisms. The disease has long been considered as a purely motor pathology that associates three symptoms: akinesia/bradykinesia (difficulty initiating movement and slowing down movement), rigidity, and tremor (which despite its association with the disease in modern folklore, affects only 30 per cent of patients).

In the last decade or so, improvements in the management of motor symptoms using pharmacological and surgical approaches has drawn the attention of clinicians to cognitive impairments, which are much more important and appear much earlier than initially thought.[9] As an emblematic disease of the basal ganglia, Parkinson's disease has played a fundamental role in our understanding of the function of the telencephalic loop. Physiological and pathophysiological approaches feed each other.

Our theoretical approach was originally designed to explain the pathophysiology of Parkinson's disease. It relies on a property of dopamine release that we have discussed only very briefly so far: volume transmission (see Chapter 6). Dopaminergic neurons maintain a constant dopamine concentration in the striatum. This constant concentration—over which the phasic responses to the presentation of stimuli and which convey the temporal difference signal

[6] Parkinson (1817).
[7] Agid (1991).
[8] Hornykiewicz (1966, 1974).
[9] Obeso et al. (2014).

is superimposed—plays an important role in regulating the gain of cortico-striatal synapses, which therefore influences G+, the total gain of the positive feedback channel (see Fig. 19.1). The drop in dopamine concentration in Parkinson's disease leads to a decrease in the gain of cortico-striatal connections and modifies the overall properties of the telencephalic loop, which is no longer able to select one module over another. The system is blocked: the subject cannot move because his motor circuit is no longer able to 'choose' one movement over another.

The cognitive impairments described in patients with Parkinson's disease can be explained by the same mechanisms but applied to prefrontal or orbito-frontal circuits. Our connectionist model allows us not only to reproduce the motor symptoms, but also the dysfunctions highlighted by pathophysiological studies. We can replicate with the model the changes in the mode of discharge, frequency, and coding of information by the neurons in the different structures of the motor circuit which have been demonstrated during almost half a century of study on the disease, both in humans or using animal models.[10]

The Deep Brain Stimulation Paradox

For a long time, there appeared to be a contradiction between the fact that the telencephalic loop is involved in decision-making and clinical observations. Lesion or disruption by deep brain stimulation (DBS) of the GPi has been used for various therapeutic purposes, ranging from the improvement of dystonia to the treatment of Tourette's syndrome. None of these approaches has reported any severe impairment in goal-oriented or automatic movement. But the model I have developed throughout this book solves the above conundrum: the basal ganglia play a critical role in the deliberative process that underlies learning, but they are not necessary for the expression of routine movements. It makes sense, therefore, that jamming the basal ganglia feedback in patients that have already learnt all the cognitive and motor skills they need in their daily lives, has no easily observable effect.[11] However, our approach predicts that after pallidotomy or during stimulation, patients should have difficulty with complex decision-making processes or learning new goal-oriented behaviours. Some preliminary experimental data seem to confirm these effects.[12]

[10] Boraud et al. (2001, 2002); Boraud et al. (2005); Leblois (2006); Leblois et al. (2006); Guthrie et al. (2013).

[11] Piron et al. (2016); Topalidou et al. (2018).

[12] Sage et al. (2003); Obeso et al. (2009).

Hyperdopaminergic Syndromes

Our model also makes it possible to propose an explanation for another aspect of Parkinson's disease: the side effects of the treatments. To compensate for motor deficits, patients are given either L-DOPA, which is a precursor of dopamine, or dopamine agonists. Due to reasons of sensitivity or overdose, these treatments can result in some surprising side effects: hyperactivity, hypersexuality, compulsive disorders, and various addictions, for example.[13] We propose to attribute to these symptoms an origin similar to that of OCD (see Fig. 19.1). The increase in the concentration of dopaminergic agonists acts as extra-synaptic dopamine at the orbitofrontal and prefrontal circuits and modifies the cortico-striatal gain. The system switches to the inappropriate selection of compulsive and inappropriate behaviours.

After a honeymoon period of five to ten years, L-DOPA, for its part, causes the appearance of repetitive involuntary movements called dyskinesia.[14] Here again, our approach proposes to explain these by permanent modifications of the cortico-striatal gain on the motor circuit, which leads to the involuntary selection of motor sequences. What we do not explain, however, are the reasons why these side effects are expressed preferentially on some circuits rather than others and have such a variability of expression from one patient to another. These reasons deserve to be explored but go beyond the scope of this book.

It is perhaps ultimately in the pathophysiology that our approach gives the full measure of its interest. It is true that our original approach was aimed at explaining the motor mechanisms of Parkinson's disease. Since our approach has become generalized to decision-making processes, dialogue with the clinical field has never totally broken. Modelling the dynamic properties of the telencephalic loop allows us to simulate pathological processes when they are known and to check how the system responds to these changes. Predictions from this theoretical approach have been confirmed so far in Parkinson's disease, a motor disease, which becomes a decision-making deficit in the broad sense. It remains to be verified that this is also the case for other pathologies. This is not trivial because we do not have experimental models of other diseases as effective as the one we have for Parkinson's disease. It would be necessary to collect the neural correlates of the pathology in humans, which is problematic for obvious ethical reasons.

[13] Thobois et al. (2010).
[14] Rascol (2000).

20
Free Will?[1]

Introduction

Are we making our decisions freely? Neuroscientists are often questioned about free will and, because I am identified as a 'specialist' in the neurobiology of decision-making, it also happens to me more than I have probably warranted.

The Libet's Paradigm

To answer this question, we first need to define 'free will'. I borrow the simplest definition from Descartes: 'the power to elect and the freedom to choose'.[2] In other words, the ability to choose independently from any exogenous determinations. Neuroscience addresses this question from a deterministic point of view.[3] The seminal experiment on this subject was proposed by Benjamin Libet in the early eighties.[4] His aim was indeed to highlight that free will is only an illusion. The experiment involves asking a subject to follow the movement of a needle on a stopwatch. The experimenter asks the subject to raise his hand when he wishes, and to note the exact moment when he became aware

[1] I am indebted to Cedric Brun for discussion regarding this chapter.
[2] Descartes (1658).
[3] I will not enter here into the debate around the possibility to naturalize free will that has animated philosophy since David Hume.
[4] Libet (1999).

How the Brain Makes Decisions. Thomas Boraud, Oxford University Press (2020). © Oxford University Press.
DOI: 10.1093/oso/9780198824367.001.0001.

of forming the intention. The subject is paired with an electroencephalogram recording. The experiment showed that the cerebral activity of the subject, in relation to the movement, changes before the subject is actually aware of his will to perform movement. Libet concluded that he had demonstrated the illusion of free will.

More recently, Soon and colleagues[5] tried to modernize this experiment using a fMRI paradigm in which the subjects had to perform voluntary additions or subtractions on sets of numbers that were proposed to them. This experiment showed that the changes in brain activity anticipated the choice made by the subject by several seconds, and they concluded that 'the brain chose before they did'.

Conceptual Misleads

However, both experiments present several flaws that make the interpretation less clear-cut than inferred by Libet and his followers. First, they were framed in a way that no other outcome was possible. In a determinist framework, how can a conscious concept not be associated with an electrophysiological activity? How can we choose before our brain? We know now that a decision emerges from competition mechanisms that are necessarily activated before the divergence point i.e. the decision per se. Therefore, a modification in brain activity must be registered before the decision itself and a fortiori the consciousness of the act.

For a long time, neurobiologists of decision-making tried to get rid of conscious processes by working with animals or doing subliminal experiments.[6] This tradition goes back to the beginning of experimental psychology;[7] the main reason for it being that subjective experience is notoriously decorrelated from the real behaviour of the subject. This cautious approach avoided being misled by framing effects such as Libet's experiment. However, it has been less scrupulously respected in recent decades.[8] Besides the experiments about free will per se and the growing interest in the neurobiology of decision-making, which was originally limited to the study of preferences and the decision-making process in uncertainty, the field has progressively broadened out to

[5] Soon et al. (2013).

[6] Pessiglione et al. (2008).

[7] See Chapter 1, note 21.

[8] The ability to carry out experiments with humans thanks to fMRI probably played a role in this evolution.

include complex behaviours that imply conscious processes, such as theory of mind and moral judgement, etc. While many of these studies engender valuable knowledge about the evolutionary roots of these processes, we should be vigilant to the boundaries of the conclusions we can draw from them, and not go too far in extrapolation. The question of whether my brain chose before me cannot be addressed because I am my brain.[9]

While neuroscience has not convincingly addressed the question of free will up until now, it is legitimate to question the relevance of this discipline to do so. It is possible to study the causal relationship between a neuronal electrical activity, even complex and basic behaviours such as movement, perception, spatial orientation, or simple choices between a few options, if the dimensions of the problems can be reduced to a handful of scalable parameters by getting rid of conscious processes. For higher-level concepts such as agency, intentionality, or free will, we can no longer neglect consciousness, and as long as nobody succeeds in reducing consciousness to a handful of measurable parameters,[10] we will not be able to operationalize the concept satisfactorily.

There is another major flaw in the design of experiments about free will, which is the blurring of the lines between agency and intentionality. Agency is related to who is at the origin of the action. Intentionality is related to the consciousness of acting and therefore is directedly related to moral responsibility. What Libet and his followers demonstrated is that a subject can be the actor of an action (he moves when his brain decides to move), but this agency reaches his consciousness later. The behaviour parameter actually considered is not so much the introspective report of the intention (intentionality) as the causality itself (agency).[11]

Back to Philosophy

More than half a century ago, Louis de Broglie pointed out that 'Many scientists have tried to make determinism and complementarity the basis of conclusions that seem to me weak and dangerous; for instance, they have used Heisenberg's uncertainty principle to bolster up human free will, though his

[9] To be more precise, the brain is a determinant part of what defines the self. The interactions between the brain and the rest of the body, the environment (including microbiotas), and surrounding society are also important components.

[10] Some try with limited success! A curious reader can have a look at Seth et al. (2006). I have to confess that I am far from being convinced!

[11] Brass et al. (2019).

principle, which applies exclusively to the behaviour of electrons and is the direct result of microphysical measurement techniques, has nothing to do with human freedom of choice. It is far safer and wiser that the physicist remains on the solid ground of theoretical physics itself and eschews the shifting sands of philosophic extrapolations.'[12] With a few adaptations, it is tempting to promulgate the same statement about neuroscience and free will.

For philosophers, indeed, the intuition of the necessity of free will is a prerequisite to the concept of responsibility which is the basis of sociability and of our legal, political, and moral system. Despite this, philosophers did not wait for Libet to undermine the concept. For instance, for Spinoza, 'only men are aware of their appetites and do not know the causes that determine them'.[13] But then compatibilist positions emerged after him such as Hobbes[14] or more recently Dennett.[15] They consist in combining the agency of the subjects and the thesis of determinism. To act freely means that our decisions are the products of external influences but they are our own external influences and they are not constrained by an external will. The debates seemed to close at this point. Paradoxically, the tentativeness of neuroscience to tackle this problem, even if inconclusive, has helped to clarify the philosophical debate. The controversy raised around the experiments of Libet and his followers allowed us to differentiate between agency and intentionality, something that philosophers didn't clearly perceive before and which has importantly helped us to refine the concepts. The legitimacy of neuroscience in the philosophical debate about free will is thus only guaranteed if it does not claim a form of universalism.

[12] Broglie (1956).
[13] Spinoza (2000, for the consulted edition).
[14] Hobbes (1999).
[15] Dennett (1991).

21
Open Questions

Introduction

Like many theories in biology, our approach remains partly conjectural insofar as it is not immune to contradiction by new experimental facts that discredit it. For the sake of simplicity, I have also been guilty of simplifications and approximations in the text. In this chapter I would like to return to a certain number of details which I have previously, deliberately left out, but which will shed additional light now.

The Globus Pallidus Affair

The most frequent reproach for our model is that it ignores the external globus pallidus. This nucleus plays an important role in regulating the activity of all other basal ganglia nuclei on which it is massively projected and is one of the key elements of the indirect pathway (see Chapter 5, Fig. 5.1), one of the three major pathways that crosses the basal ganglia. We ignored it in our model because it simplifies the interactions and the dynamic properties of the indirect pathway and is very similar to that of the hyper-direct pathway which we modelled.[1] Introducing it into our model would not change its dynamic properties in depth (Leblois 2006). However, although it seems trivial and a little tedious, it would be necessary to confirm this conjecture, if only to dissect the conditions in which oscillations appear, which are one of the electrophysiological signatures of Parkinson's disease (see Chapter 19, Fig. 19.1).

[1] For discussion about the reason why we made this choice, see Leblois (2006); Leblois et al. (2006); Guthrie et al. (2013).

How the Brain Makes Decisions. Thomas Boraud, Oxford University Press (2020). © Oxford University Press.
DOI: 10.1093/oso/9780198824367.001.0001.

From Perception to Decision-Making

Considering the specific properties of cortical columns allows us to briefly address a substantial area of neuroscience that I have voluntarily ignored in this book up until now: perception. For those who work on sensory systems (vision, hearing, smell, etc.) the core question is 'How does the brain distinguish between two stimuli?' Researchers rely on the properties of cortical structures that they have also contributed to characterizing in large part,[2] for it is mainly neuroscientists working on vision who have shown that cortical learning is one of the basic mechanisms of the distinction between two stimuli. However, following an interesting anchoring bias, researchers working on sensory systems tend to underestimate the role of subcortical structures. They propose a theory of decision-making based on a continuum of contrast mechanisms propagating from perception to action.[3] However, in my opinion, there is a fundamental difference in distinguishing between two stimuli versus deciding between two options. In the first case it is a question of differentiating between two different inputs will be more appropriate: it is a simple matter of contrast and the cortical columns with their systems of lateral inhibition and positive feedback control are quite apt to do this. In the second case, you need an internal option generator, and this generator (noise) does not exist in cortical systems. In fact, most models of sensory systems use the cortex to increase the signal-to-noise ratio! Therefore, decision-making cannot be considered as a continuation of the perception process. This is a different process with its own dynamics.

An Emotionless Brain?

Throughout this book, I have deliberately avoided psychological considerations, adopting an approach similar to that initially advocated by experimental psychologists. As an experimentalist, it is very difficult for me to define and quantify emotions, and even moreso to identify them in animal models. I prefer to eliminate them by sticking to quantifiable scalars (such as value, utility, or expected utility). But it is difficult to talk about decision-making while ignoring the rich literature on the interactions between emotions and

[2] Shepherd (2011).
[3] Cisek (2006); Shadlen and Kiani (2013).

rationality[4] that perpetrate the old debate of the Stoics and the Epicureans. Until recently, psychologists have tended to oppose a rational and calculating 'cold' system versus an irrational and emotional 'hot' system.[5] But this segregation is not resistant to neurobiology; the human uses the same brain structures to make a decision with both serenity and under the influence of emotions.[6] Besides, showing a preference is already a form of emotion. Therefore, there are no 'cold' decisions, but simply decisions that are influenced by different kinds of emotion. These add an extra dimension by modulating the scalars (utility, hope, etc.) on which the decision-making system is based to make its choices.

If emotions reflect the imbalances of homeostasis[7] and our rationality is so limited, it would seem that neurobiology gives reason to Epicureans against Stoics: it would be better to trust his emotions (and stabilize his homeostasis) than his reason (which can easily be deceived).

[4] Including, not comprehensively: sadness (Lerner et al. 2013); regret (Coricelli et al. 2005); empathy (Andari et al. 2010); anger (Lerner and Keltner 2001; Bagneux et al. 2012); and fear (Lerner and Keltner 2001) etc.

[5] Sloman (1996); Kahneman (2012).

[6] Seymour and Dolan (2008); Lerner et al. (2014).

[7] Homeostasis is the internal balance of a biological organism. All behaviours would have as ultimate objective the conservation of this homeostasis. For some neurobiologists, emotions are signals indicating an imbalance that needs to be addressed (Vincent 1986).

22
Conclusions

Toward a Natural History of (ir)rationality

It has been barely 30 years since Schultz's, Newsome's, and Movshon's experiments. During this lapse of time, neuroscientists—consisting of anatomists, electrophysiologists, behaviourists, neurologists, and psychiatrists—joined the community of psychologists and economists who studied rationality. Together, they were able to set up experimental paradigms to try to better understand the neurobiological foundations of the learning and decision-making processes (and, incidentally, to define their limits). The conceptual framework defined by all of these paradigms has been called neuroeconomics. Neuroeconomics is therefore the study of the neural correlates of rationality. As such, this book can be considered as an essay on neuroeconomics, but its originality lies in the approach I have adopted.

The classical neuroeconomic approach begins with an axiomatic postulate assuming that 'such a process is described by such equation(s)' and then seeks a neural correlate to the equation(s) during a task that combines a process of learning and decision-making. It is therefore a top-down approach that validates a theoretical hypothesis and highlights the structures involved. This approach, which is ultimately only an extension of those used in psychology or experimental economics, to which an additional layer of neurobiological parameters has been added, has improved our knowledge, but not without its pitfalls. i) It is correlative and observing that the neural activity of a structure correlated with an algorithm does not necessarily imply that this structure is directly responsible for the underlying process.[1] ii) The algorithm itself has only a descriptive value, it is not informative about how the process is performed by the neural population. iii) The theoretical argument generally reflects the beliefs of the author, usually with a more or less assumed teleologic background (see Chapter 10).

[1] This remark is true for France but does not stand for the UK or the US where pharmacological manipulation can be performed in healthy volunteers. See for the record a British study confirming the role of dopamine in learning processes (Pessiglione et al. 2006).

How the Brain Makes Decisions. Thomas Boraud, Oxford University Press (2020). © Oxford University Press.
DOI: 10.1093/oso/9780198824367.001.0001.

In humans, these studies are conducted using fMRI. This method makes it possible to measure a global signal but does not provide information on its exact nature, and the spatial and temporal resolutions are limited. It also results in an overrepresentation of the role of the cortex compared to deep nuclei whose total volume rarely exceeds a handful of voxels. It thus leads us to neglect the role of the latter in comparison to the former.

The dominant theories of neuroeconomics are heavily influenced by machine learning. Thus they tend to dissociate the process of decision-making (the actor) from that of evaluation (the critic) whereas the experimental paradigms used generally amalgamate the two processes. If we take the example of the two-armed bandit task, when the values are initially unknown, the learning and decision-making processes depend on each other and it becomes difficult to determine if the subject does not optimize because their learning is incomplete or their decision-making process is deficient.

Our bottom-up approach makes it possible to overcome a number of these pitfalls. In posing our initial question: 'How does a neural substrate decide?', we built a decision-making structure from less than a dozen elementary units: the diachetron (see Appendix A).

We then showed that it is possible to give our system a learning rule from very simple biological processes (the three-component Hebbian rule). This allowed us to show that what we called the diencephalic and telencephalic loops had a structure very close to the minimum decision-making machine and that dopamine gave them the ability to learn. We concluded that decision-making processes were governed by a combination of stochastic mechanisms and divergent processes: a small random variation at the time of decision-making could cause a switch from one option to another. Noise is one of the essential features of the system that allows it to decide when there is no clear preference that emerges, but suddenly, this results in a sub-optimal behaviour in economic terms. This sub-optimality may also be an evolutionary advantage since it makes it possible to explore an environment spontaneously and thus to assess if the contingency rules are evolving.

As evolution progressed, the development of the cortex increased the number of possible behaviours and offered a greater diversity of options among which this elementary system worked. This development was accompanied by a complexification and a hierarchization, which produced the capacity to build mental representations and allowed us to anticipate. But since this system is not a de novo structure, the initial limitations persist and the presence of noise may explain some of the limitations of human rationality. Other limits are a by-product of the development of the cortex. It allows the emergence of automatic processes that are necessary for skill acquisition and habitual behaviours, but these automatic processes also underlie some of the heuristics (such as false beliefs, anchoring, halo, etc.).

Our approach is not exclusive. We have shown that it is compatible with the algorithms of the automatic approach, even if the underlying symbolism (the actor-critic model) is to be handled with caution. It also provides a substrate for the phenomena highlighted by behavioural economists such as heuristics or the dilution effect. These last explanations are conjectural and would need to be analysed in more detail. Finally, our connectionist model has a significant explanatory value with regard to the pathophysiology of decision-making processes.

This approach also provides new pathways to explore different areas. By addressing the problem of rationality from a dual connectionist and evolutionist perspective, it highlights that our brain is not capable of producing a purely rational process. The selection mechanisms that have governed the evolution of the central nervous system of vertebrates from lamprey to human have not been able to completely erase the intrinsic element of chance in the decision-making process. *Homo sapiens* is not 'programmed' to be a *homo logicus* as our Western culture would have us believe. If this is so it may be simply because pure logic is not an evolutionary edge and there is more interest in keeping a limited rationality than an absolute one.

When one sees the totalitarian drifting to which society, based on absolute rationality, may lead, it is legitimate to think that a little irrationality does not hurt.

Acknowledgements

First of all, I would like to express my gratitude to David Hansel and Arthur Leblois, with whom this adventure began and who are both behind the theoretical formalization that I have only taken up and developed. Collaborating with you is always a pleasure and an enrichment. Thank you, Comrades!

A special mention to Peter Redgrave who drew my attention to the evolutionist dimension in 2006. My approach owes a lot to him, for that he is thanked here.

I would also like to express my gratitude to all the students and postdocs who worked on the projects that underpin this approach: Benjamin Pasquereau, Agnès Nadjar, Cyril Dejean, Steeve Laquitaine, Berangere Ballion, Martin Guthrie, Camille Piron, Brice de la Crompe, Daisuke Kase, Meropi Topalidou, Aurelien Nioche, Marc Deffains, Basile Garcia, Marie Penavayre, and Aude Retailleau. Without you nothing could have been done. Some of you have already become accomplished researchers and I am sure that others will not fail to become so. I wish you a long and happy career and I hope that we will continue to have fun together.

To my other playfellows with whom we have exchanged points of view, ideas, equations of the world, arguments (if not there is no debate), many glasses and sometimes fruitful collaborations: Erwan Bezard, François and Francesca Ichas, Wassilios Meissner, Hamid Benazzouz, Rony Paz, Genela Morris, Nicolas Mallet, Sacha Bourgeois-Gironde, Stephane Charpier, Christelle Baunez, Laurent Venance, Pierre-Olivier 'POF' Fernagut, Francois Gonon, Mathias Pessiglione, Mehdi Khamassi, Nicolas Rougier, Catherine Le Moine, Philippe De Deurweardere, André Garenne, Pierre Burbaud, Dominique Guehl, Frederic Alexandre, Paolo Gubellini, Pete Magill, Andy Sharrot, Yonatan Loewenstein, Jose Obeso, Atsushi Nambu, Philippe Vernier, Suzana Herculano-Houzel, Sten Grillner, Carole Levenes, Greg Porras, Aline Desmet, Anastasia Christakou, Thomas Michelet, Jean-Marie Cabelguen, Sebastien Bouret, Anna Beyeler, Estelle Mallet, Cédric Brun as well as most of those whose work I quote in these pages.

I would also like to thank my masters under whose auspices I have trained and who have watched over my career as benevolent *Parcae* since my recruitment at the CNRS: Christian Gross, Bernard Bioulac, and Hagai Bergman.

I thank, of course, Delphine, Theophile, and Virgile who have always been a steadfast support to me and the rest of my family who are kind enough to make me believe that what I tell them interests them while my activities compared to theirs often seem a bit abstruse.

I would like to end with a special mention for my own personal text editor, her critical review and proof editing, performed with humour, avoided me appearing too ludicrous with my approximate spelling.

APPENDIX A

The Diachetron

In order to illustrate the principles explained in Chapter 4, this Appendix proposes to design a decision-making machine that must choose between two options on demand. Let us specify our requirements: this imaginary organism, which we will call a Diachetron,[1] must operate on biological principles with the most economical nervous system.

The Motor System

To be able to express a choice, our system is made of two motor units (Units 1 and 2) that allow it to perform two different actions (Action 1 and 2) and two excitatory motor neurons (neuron M1 and neuron M2), which activate Units 1 and 2 respectively. If the M1 neuron fires at a frequency greater than an activation threshold, which we arbitrarily chose to be equal to 10 spikes, it activates Unit 1 which performs Action 1. In a similar way, if the neuron M2 fires at a frequency greater than or equal to 10 spikes, it activates Unit 2, which performs Action 2.

In order to transmit our request to make a decision, we must add a sensory system. It will be minimalist: a simple sensory neuron S that transforms an external stimulus (our request) into a train of spikes. This neuron will be excitatory and connected to M1 and M2 by connections with an identical gain. When a stimulus is applied, it activates them in a similar way. To make this simple and economical (in real biological systems, the production of a spike has a significant energy cost) we will consider that our three neurons are phasic. Their intrinsic discharge frequency is zero, so they produce action potentials only if they are activated. Our Diachetron looks for now as in Fig. A1.

Our problem now boils down to activating one of the two motor neurons and keeping the other one below the threshold.

A first possibility is to activate them differentially by external stimuli. However, this is cheating since the decision is no longer made by our Diachetron, but by an outside intervention. The solution must come from within.

A second solution would be that when applying a stimulus on the neuron S, one of the two motor neurons has a discharge frequency always higher than the threshold and the other always lower. This could be achieved by assigning different gains to the S-M1 and S-M2 coupling. But again, there would be no real decision-making here, since our imaginary organism would always choose the same action. In fact, for the Diachetron to decide for itself, we cannot economize the interaction between neurons A and B.

The Decision-Making System

A glance at the literature confirms that the simplest system to obtain an imbalance between two neurons subjected to the same activation consists of two inhibitory neurons. We will therefore add A1 and A2, two inhibitory neurons, coupled reciprocally and symmetrically. So, if A1 is activated, it inhibits A2 and vice versa. For the sake of simplicity and economy,

[1] Purists will forgive my dog Greek.

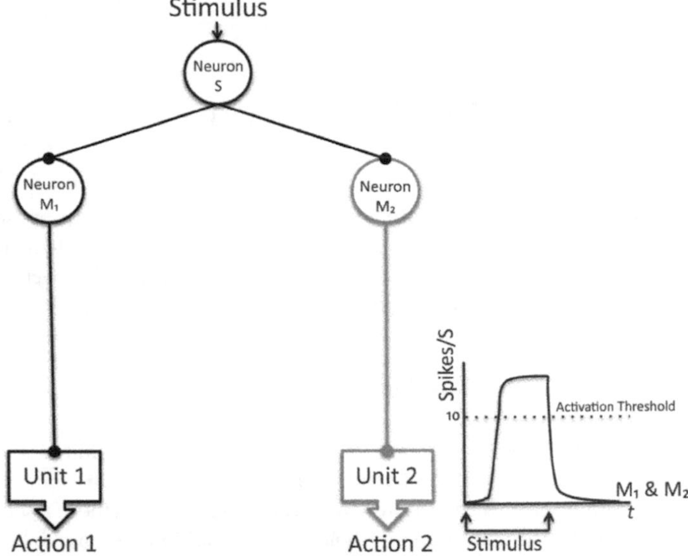

Fig. A1 First step of the Diachetron, the motor system. S, M1 and M2 neurons are excitatory. A stimulus applied on S leads to an identical response of M1 and M2. There is no choice since the two units pass the threshold (dashed line).

these neurons will also be phasic. In the jargon of neuroscientists these two neurons exert lateral inhibition on each other. We connect our decision-making system to the motor system with symmetrical inputs: M1 coupling with A1 and M2 with A2. This results in a very stable architecture, A1 and A2 mutually inhibiting each other. Our decision-making system is not yet able to activate one of the two populations in a differential way. For this, we will have to involve an additional property: noise.

We will add a Gaussian noise B of 0.05 variance into neurons A1 and A2 of our Diachetron.[2] It means that the variance in the distribution of spike occurrences of these neurons is 5 per cent higher than that of a Poisson process, which is physiologically quite acceptable. Thus, identical activation will induce a slightly different response from A1 and A2 neurons. This difference is sufficient to break the balance and the activation state of the two neurons will diverge: one will be activated, the other will remain silent (Fig. A2). However, the system is relatively unstable: it can alternate from one state to another without modification of the stimulus. If the noise is too large, it can also be triggered in the absence of a stimulus, which is not in our specifications. It will therefore be necessary to find a solution to stabilize it. We will come back to this.

The Coupling

We will now re-connect our decision-making system to our motor system so the latter benefits from the divergence between A1 and A2. We could save extra neurons by the feedback

[2] A Gaussian noise is a stochastic process of which distribution follows a Gaussian law with a zero mean. In the case of our artificial neurons, this will cause a modification of the firing probability of our neuron as follows: $P'(t) = B + P(t)$ if $B + P(t) \geq 0$ or $P'(t) = 0$ if $B + P(t) < 0$. $P(t) = 1 / F$; F is the average mean firing rate of the neuron reduced to the time scale t; and B has a Gaussian distribution with mean=0 and variance=0.05 (for a noise at 5 per cent).

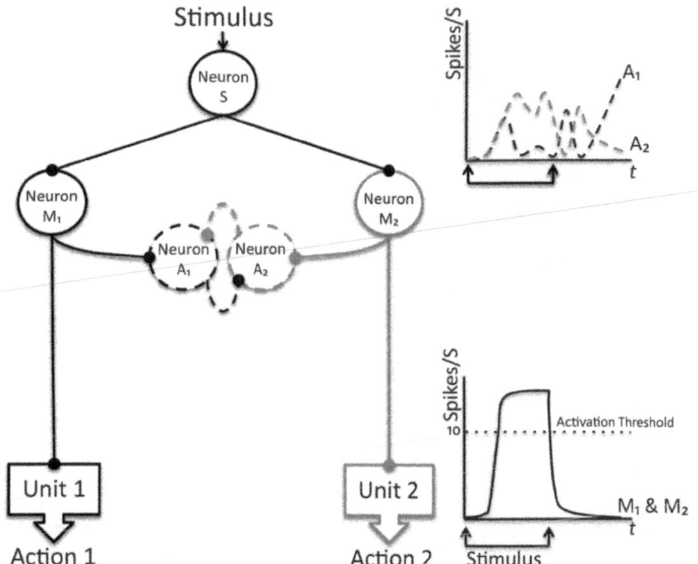

Fig. A2 Second step of the Diachetron, the decision-making system. A1 and A2 neurons are inhibitory. The presence of noise makes the A1-A2 system unstable. When a stimulus is applied to S, the system diverges after a certain lapse of time despite identical excitation by the M1-A1 and M2-A2 couplings: when one of A1 or A2 is activated, the other one is inhibited. Note that the system is unstable and switches from one state to another, sometimes even in the absence of a stimulus. Note also that in the absence of feedback on M1 and M2, the response of A1 and A2 does not change with respect to the configuration.

couplings A1-M1 and A2-M2, but this solution, despite its elegance, does not work because it creates what is called a negative feedback loop on M1 neurons and M2: when activated, they receive equivalent inhibition, stabilizing them in an inactivated state.

We will now add two inhibitory neurons A'1 and A'2 between neurons A and M. A1 is coupled with A'1 which is coupled with M1. The architecture is symmetrical with respect to A2, A'2, and M2. For the system to work, we have to make sure that the neurons A' are tonic and have a non-zero basal activity (say 10 spikes). There are several reasons for this, the most intuitive being that it has to operate in two directions. Thus, if the A neuron is activated, the frequency of A' decreases (see the example in Fig. A3). If its initial discharge frequency was zero, the activation of A would have no effect on A'. This architecture also solves the stability problem that we encountered with the previous configuration (Fig. A2).

The A1-A'1-M1 and A2-A'2-M2 complexes form positive feedback control loops: the synapses function as algebraic operators; two successive inhibitory synapses have the same effects as an activating synapse ($-1 \times -1 = 1$). This means that the neurons A1 and A2 exert an activating influence on themselves, amplifying the effects of an imbalance between the two neurons as they occur. The divergence between A1 and A2 will be faster and amplified. It will remain as long as the stimulus lasts. In addition, the negative tonus of neuron A', when no stimulus occurs, will act as a filter, which will maintain the inactive system by preventing an imbalance appearing in the absence of a stimulus.

Let's summarize the dynamics of our network at this point (see Fig. A3).

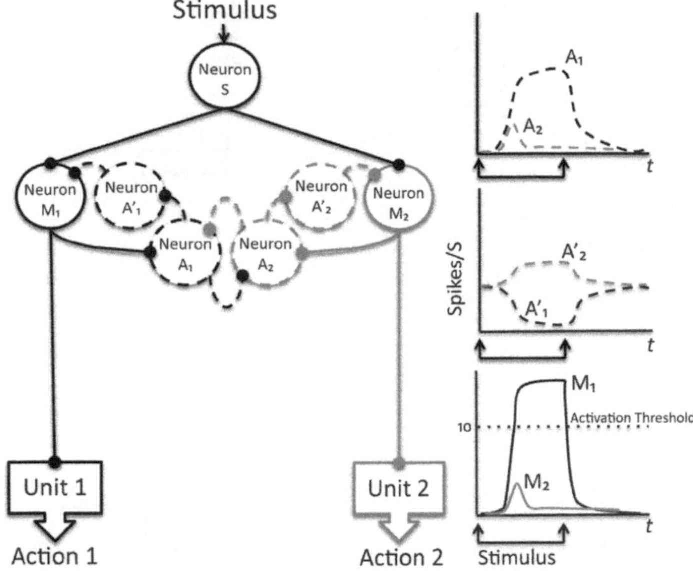

Fig. A3 Third step of the Diachetron, the coupling. When we apply a stimulus on S, the system diverges. In our example, A1 wins the competition (but in 50 per cent of the cases it will be A2). A'1 and A'2 transmit this divergence to M1 and M2 and help to amplify and stabilize the divergence. M1 goes well above the threshold (dashed line) while M2 is inhibited. It took us seven neurons to run our Diachetron.

- At rest (without external stimulation) our system is silent (no neurons produce action potentials), the effects of noise are filtered by A'1 and A'2.
- When a stimulus activates the neuron S, the noise causes an imbalance between A1 and A2 which is amplified by the positive feedback loop A-A'-M-A. This results in an explosive decoupling of the activity of the neurons A, A', and M. Thus, a differential activation of Units 1 and 2 is obtained. The system chooses one of the two actions randomly, with identical probability.
- When the stimulus is stopped, the system returns to its resting state, thanks to the inhibitory drive exerted by A' neurons on M neurons.

The Diachetron: A Dumb Decision-Making Engine . . .

We fulfilled our specifications with only seven neurons. This seems to be the minimum number for a virtual neural network that can choose between two options.[3] Since our

[3] For comparison, one of the smallest known neural networks is the nervous system of the *Caenorhabditis Elegans*, a small worm broadly used in science because its genome and physiology have been fully mapped. It consists of 279 neurons, of which only 90 belong to the decision-making system (Jarrell et al. 2012).

system is symmetrical, it has a 50 per cent chance of choosing the A1 action and a 50 per cent chance of choosing the A2 action.

It is therefore not possible to determine a priori which action will be chosen. An acrimonious reader might wonder why we struggled to invent such a complex device, replete with a mouthful of a name and making decisions at random, while the 'executive decision-maker' of Brazil (see Chapter 2, Fig. 2.2) would have solved any conflict between two options more elegantly? To answer this question, we will have to push our logic a little further.

For a Decision To Be Relevant, the Question Asked Must Be Relevant

For now, the actions A1 and A2 that our Diachetron is able to perform are abstract and equivalent. It is therefore perfectly justified to choose one or the other without any preference. Let us now transform the environment of our imaginary organism. We will now decide that one of the actions has a positive outcome: it brings a reward to our organism. The nature of this reward remains abstract for the moment. If desired, the reader can put here whatever motivates him the most at the time of reading (food, drink, sex, money, social status, etc.). The other option is neutral (no outcome). We will assign an arbitrary value of 1 to the option that provides the reward and 0 to the option that provides nothing. The difficulty of the task is that we do not know which one is the most interesting. The system will have to learn this on its own. For this, we will use neural plasticity rules.

The Learning Process

In the late 1940s, neuropsychologist Donald Hebb stated the rule that bears his name and can be summarized as follows:[4] if a neuron A is connected by a synapse to a neuron B and the two neurons increase their activity together, then the gain of the synapse that connects them will be increased. So, when neuron A will be excited again, the response of neuron B will be amplified. It will take 20 years for the underlying mechanism to be demonstrated in the hippocampus by Lømo[5] in the form of what he called long-term potentiation (LTP): a gradual increase in response from a post-synaptic neuron to the excitation of the pre-synaptic neuron that persists over time. Hebbian learning and LTP form the basis of learning processes in the nervous system.

To help our system to decide in a relevant way, it is necessary to strengthen the coupling between the neurons M and A associated with the action of value 1 (that which is rewarded) by Hebbian learning. Since it does not know which one it is (and also because the environment may change, but we will come back to this), the system must be symmetrical. Finally, it is necessary to inform the system if a reward is provided. We will then start by adding a neuron R which is sensitive to the reward. This is our second 'sensory' neuron, that is to say that it informs the Diachetron about its interactions with the environment. This neuron is phasic and excitatory. If the action provides a reward, it is activated for a short time, otherwise it remains silent.

It is then necessary to condition the Hebbian learning at the M-A synapse to the presence of the reward, when provided. We will use an additional neuron (C). It will have a property

[4] Hebb (1949).

[5] Anderson and Lømo (1966).

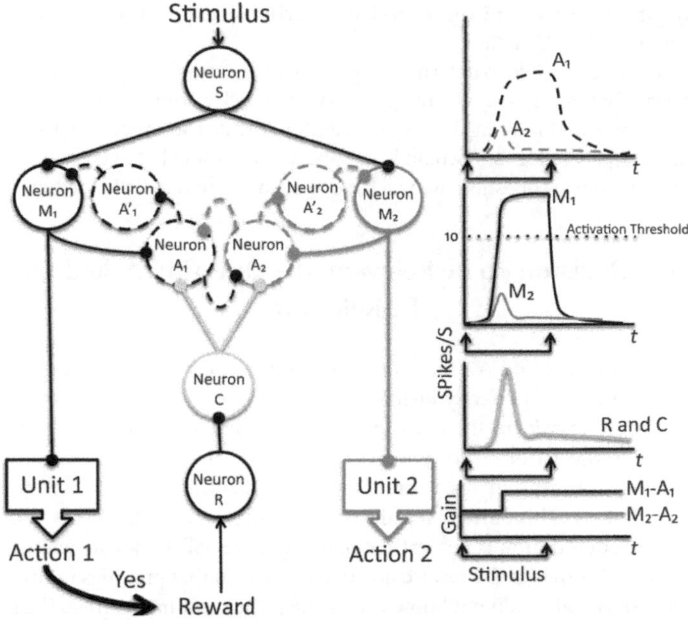

Fig. A4 Fourth step of the Diachetron, the learning system. In this example, the selected action causes a reward (here it is Action 1). Activation of the modulator neuron C reinforces the coupling M1-A1 because these two neurons are activated, but not the coupling M2-A2, with these two neurons being rapidly inactivated.

that differentiates it from other neurons in the system: it will be a neuromodulator. If it increases its activity, it does not change that of the post-synaptic neuron, but enhances the gain of co-activated synapses. This results in tri-component Hebbian learning. We will then couple neuron R to neuron C and neuron C to neurons A1 and A2 (see Fig. A4).

Thus, when one of the two actions result in a reward, the neuron R activates the neuron C which reinforces only the coupling between the two neurons corresponding to the selected action. The gain between the two activated neurons will change from an average state to a high state. The difference in gain between M1-A1 and M2-A2 is such that from now on the Diachetron will choose the rewarded action more often or even exclusively (see Fig. A5). For the price of two additional neurons, we have equipped our Diachetron with a learning ability. The 'executive decision-maker' is no longer random! Our system is able to optimize its behaviour without outside intervention.

A Too Well Adapted Engine

In our specifications, the Diachetron is now optimized, but this optimization is associated with a certain weakness: if by chance the context changes and the action associated with a reward is reversed suddenly, the Diachetron is no longer able to readjust. For this, we must introduce a devaluation mechanism for a chosen option if it is no longer rewarded. The simplest solution would be to add a mechanism for decreasing the M-A gain if an option is

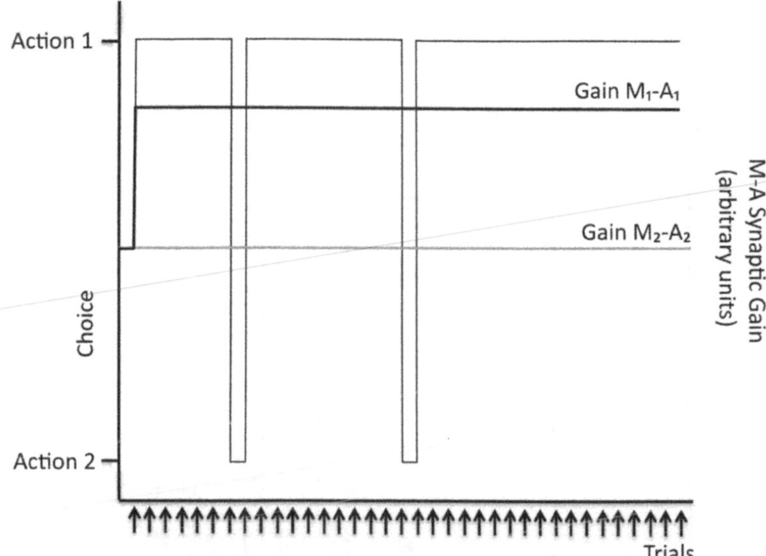

Fig. A5 Reinforcement learning (tri-component Hebbian learning). The thin continuous curve shows discrete choice of the Diachetron between Action 1 (top) and Action 2 (bottom) at each new trial (stimulus-response combination, shown by an arrow below the x axis) for the configuration represented in Fig. A4 (Action 1 rewarded). The gain of the M1-A1 coupling increases when the system is rewarded for the first time thus biasing the competition between A1 and A2 toward the former. As a result, Action 1 is consequently chosen most often. However, residual noise leads from time to time to the choice of Action 2.

chosen and not rewarded. The mechanisms for this type of solution exist in nature; they are grouped under the term extinction.

Among these mechanisms, we will focus on the mirror mechanism of LTP: long-term depression (aka anti-Hebbian learning), which causes two neurons that fire together under certain conditions to reduce their synaptic coupling. It is therefore perfectly legitimate to consider decreasing the gain of M-A if neuron C is no longer activated for a given action. We thus maintain the same network as for Fig. A4, but we add this anti-Hebbian process, which decreases the gain of the pair M-A corresponding to the unrequited action (Fig. A6). Thus, if we apply a change of condition after 20 tests, for example, it will quickly readjust to this new situation.

The Two-Armed Bandit Strikes Again

Our system is able to learn, unlearn, and re-learn in an environment whose contingency rules change. However, in the real world, our actions are not always rewarded in a binary way, because a certain degree of uncertainty still persists. Let's consider the case of the predator who charges at its prey: the latter can dodge at the last moment and thus postpone its

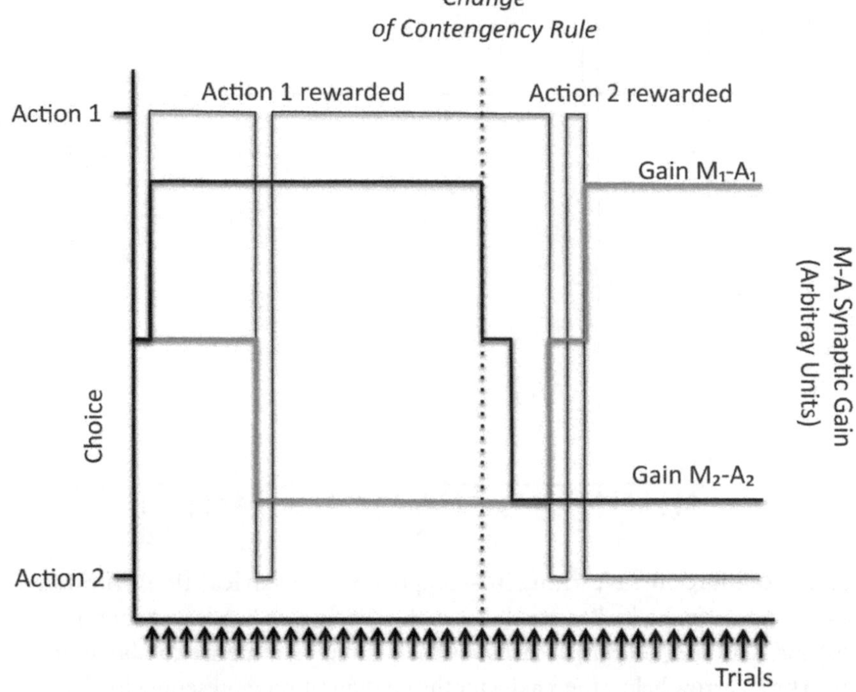

Fig. A6 Anti-Hebbian learning. The gain of the coupling M1-A1 increases in the same way as in the previous condition. On the other hand, the gain of M2-A2 decreases the first time the system chooses Action 2 and is not rewarded. This mechanism further reinforces the bias in favour of choosing Action 1. When the contingency rule changes after 20 tries and Action 2 is rewarded, the system relearns quickly.

fate for a while. It will therefore be interesting to test our Diachetron in an uncertain environment in order to validate its ability to adapt to the contingencies of a more ecological environment. As we saw in Chapter 1, behaviourists use the two-armed bandit paradigm to address the concept of uncertainty. It consists of asking a subject to choose between two options of different probability of reward (P_r). These contingencies are covert at the beginning of the test (see Fig. 1.2).

The reader will intuitively understand that if we submit our Diachetron to such a protocol, it will have difficulty learning the respective values of each option since the M-A and A-C couplings will vary according to the administration of the reward.[6] For the system to improve its performance during learning, it is necessary to find a way to maintain a long-term memory of the consequences of the different actions performed. Again, the solution

[6] In fact, his behaviour will be close to the 'win-stay, loose-switch' strategy sometimes described in the literature. However, here, it will not be purely of this type because of the noise that persists in the activity of neuron A and which can still favour an action whose coupling M-A is not the most important.

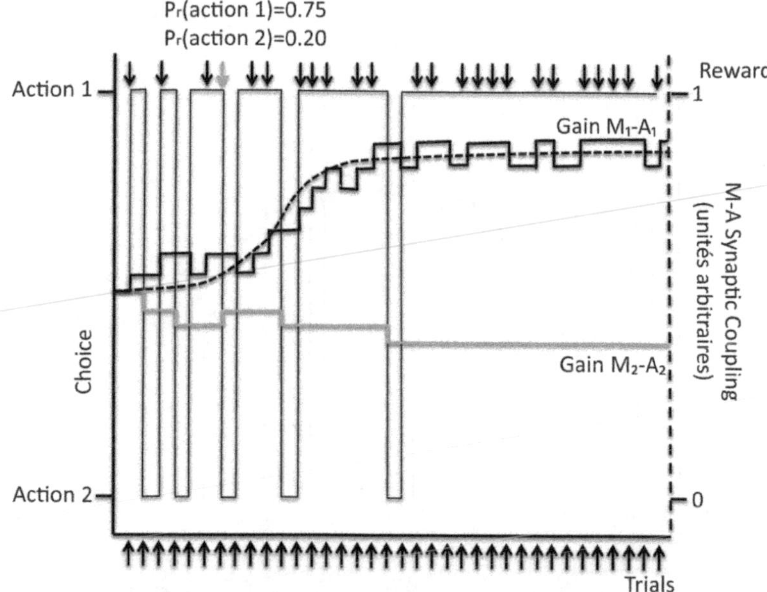

Fig. A7 The two-armed bandit task. In our example, Action 1 is rewarded three times out of four and Action 2 one time out of five. The gain of the two A-M couplings evolves gradually in stages according to the choices and rewards represented by the arrows at the top (in black when Action 1 is rewarded and in grey when Action 2 is rewarded). The coupling gain increases or decreases until an arbitrary threshold (which we introduced for the sake of plausibility). The dotted curve represents the probability that the system chooses Action 1 based on the previous choices. It is commonly known as the learning curve. Note that for our Diachetron, its kinetics are similar to those of the M1-A1 gain.

is simple and does not require additional neurons. It is enough to slightly modify the properties of the coupling of neurons M and A (see Fig. A7). We are going to make sure that this coupling can have several levels and be reinforced gradually each time a reward is administered, thus preserving a memory of the previous choices. In order to remain in a physiologically plausible domain, the gain between two neurons cannot vary infinitely and will be bounded between zero and a maximum value.[7] If P_r(Action 1) and P_r(Action 2) varies, the system is able to detect and adapt (see Fig. A8). Therefore, our initial goal is reached with nine neurons and the very simple rules of plasticity.

Our solution is far from perfect. In particular, re-adaptation to new conditions takes almost twice as long as initial learning because the system must be unlearned to re-learn new conditions. We have also neglected a certain number of constraints such as the energy expenditure required for each action, the delay that usually exists between an action and its consequences, perception problems that are here oversimplified, and so on. In short, our

[7] See Chapter 17 for a natural solution for a system to limits itself.

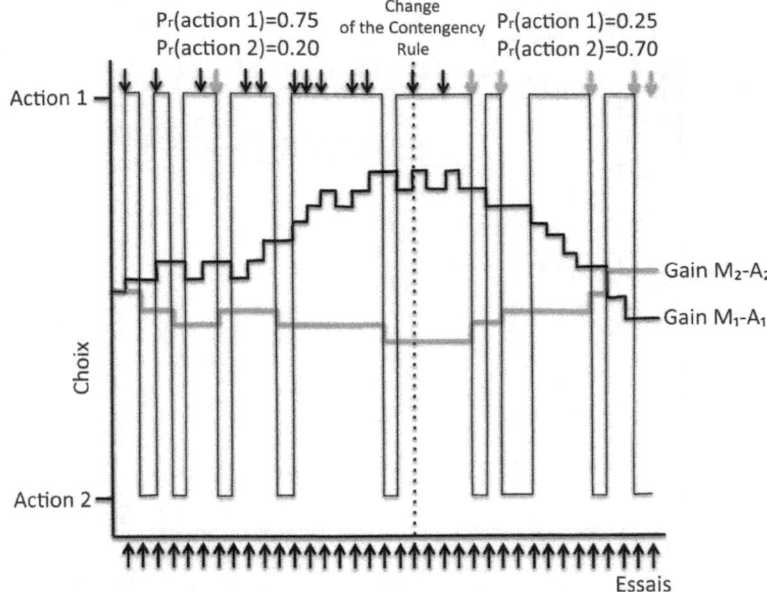

Fig. A8 Rule modifications in the two-armed bandit task. When the contingency rule is reversed, the system must first bring the gains of the M1-A1 and M2-A2 coupling to their initial values before relearning the new contingencies. The Diachetron takes time to lose his old habits and acquire new ones.

Diachetron is not likely to propel itself to the top of the evolutionary ladder, but it is honourably fulfilling the task it has been assigned to.

The Take-Home Message of the Diachetron

This long Appendix, a bit tedious I admit, allows us to identify the major mechanisms that allow the nervous system to make goal-oriented decisions. It is probably useful to summarize them now.

For a decision between two options to emerge from a neural network, an architecture consisting of at least nine neurons is required (see Fig. A4), but more importantly, it has to possess the following properties:

1. This network must have an effector system acting on the environment that sets the possible options (M1 and M2) and a system (S) that initiates the behaviour and triggers the sequence of phenomena that will allow the system to choose one of the two options.
2. To choose, a mechanism of competition is necessary so that a population is activated and the other is inhibited. The simplest is made of reciprocally connected inhibitory neurons (A1 and A2).

3. To create an imbalance and to allow the system to switch one way or the other, requires noise in the system, that is to say imperfections in the generation of the spikes.
4. The presence of noise makes the system unstable. A positive feedback mechanism helps to stabilize the system in three possible states: no choice, choice of option 1, choice of option 2 (loops A1-A'1-M1-A1 and A2-A'2 -M2-A2).

Equipped with these four principles, we obtain a system capable of choosing randomly. If we want the system to be capable of learning, two additional principles need to be integrated:

5. A system of valuation for the consequences of the action chosen (R and C): if the two options are equivalent, there is no reason to prefer one over the other.
6. Rules of learning and unlearning that allow facilitation of the appropriate decisions and a degree of plasticity if the rules of the contingencies between actions and rewards change (modification of the gain of the M-A connections).

APPENDIX B

Glossary

Acetylcholine. Main excitatory neurotransmitter of the peripheral nervous system. In the central nervous system, it is present in the striatum. A neuron that releases acetylcholine is called a cholinergic neuron.

Anamniotes. This word of Greek origin designates the lower vertebrates whose embryo is devoid of amnion: fish (in which I include agnates for the sake of simplicity) and amphibians.

Basal ganglia. Sub-cortical nuclei of telencephalic and diencephalic origin. Since the 1990s it has been customary to organize them as a three-layer system consisting of two input structures (the striatum and the subthalamic nucleus), two exit structures (the internal globus pallidus and the substantia nigra pars reticulata) and an intermediate structure (the external globus pallidus). These archaic nuclei appeared with the first vertebrates. Their organization is detailed in Chapter 5. They are one of the core elements of the decision-making and learning system.

BG. Acronym for basal ganglia.

Bifurcation. Describes a process in which a small change in a physical parameter produces a major change in the organization of the system.

BOLD signal. Abbreviation for blood-oxygen-level-dependent signal. It refers to the signal collected in fMRI. It is an indirect measure of the neuronal activity of a structure.

CA1, CA2, CA3. Abbreviations for *Corne d'Ammon* 1, 2, and 3. They are subdivisions of the hippocampus.

Central nervous system. Subdivision of the nervous system corresponding to the encephalon and the spinal cord. It computes and generates responses to stimulation of the peripheral nervous system.

Cingular loop. Subdivision of the telencephalic loop involved in close relationship with the hippocampus, in the building of a mental representation of the environment in mammals (see Figs. 17.2 and 19.1).

Coefficient of variation. In statistics, the coefficient of variation is the variance divided by the mean. Spike production is a stochastic process that is supposed to obey a Poisson distribution law, that is, its variance is equal to its mean. This is not the case in the basal ganglia (striatum and globus pallidus especially) where the coefficient of variation is significantly greater than 1. This intrinsic variability is related to the noise in the system which is one important element of decision-making processes.

Contingency. The contingency rule is the degree of association between an action and a reward. It is measured by a probability (P) between 0 and 1. It is explicit when it is known (this is the case in lotteries of economy) and implicit when it is unknown (as in the protocols of the *k*-armed bandit). In the first case, the subjects can calculate the expectation, in the second case, they must estimate it from the consequences of their choices.

Cortex. The anterior and dorsal part of the telencephalon mantle, called the pallium in anamniotes, reptiles, and birds becomes the cortex in mammals. This change of terminology corresponds to a huge increase in its surface and a change of organization. It is organized in a modular way into mini functional units made up of six layers (five in some structures such as the hippocampus) around a projection neuron (that is to say it communicates with other structures) and inter-neurons. This loosely cylindrical functional unit is called a column.

DA. Abbreviation for dopamine.

Diachetron. Dog Greek to designate the minimal decision-making engine described in Appendix A. It represents a system made up of the smallest possible number of neurons to choose between two options. It is a heuristic device that allows us to highlight the principles involved in the decision-making and learning processes.

Diencephalic loop. Network constituted by the thalamus and the basal ganglia. It is a neologism that I use in this book because there is no existing terminology to coin it. The name is not fully satisfactory because it is a network that combines elements of the diencephalon and the telencephalon. Its architecture is described in Fig. 12.1.

Diencephalon. Medial subdivision of the brain consisting of the thalamus, the subthalamic nucleus, the hypothalamus, and the epiphysis.

Direct pathway. Pathway between the cortex and the GPi that passes through the striatum. Its influence is inhibitory: its activation decreases the activity of GPi neurons (see Fig. 7.2).

Dopamine. This catecholamine is one of the main neuromodulators of the central nervous system. It is released by the neurons of the substantia nigra and the ventral tegmental area. It modulates the activity of its target neurons through two large families of receptors. It plays a key role in the learning process.

Ethogram. Also called an inventory of behaviours. It refers to the number and diversity of individual or social behaviours that a species can display.

Expected value. For a given lottery (A), the expected value E(A) = Probability × Value. This is the average of the expected gains over several repetitions (see Chapter 1). Rationality would require that between two options of different expected values, one chooses the highest one (provided one has the means to compute both of them). This is often not the case.

fMRI. Acronym commonly used as such to refer to functional magnetic resonance imaging methods.

GABA. Acronym for gamma-aminobutyric acid. It is the main inhibitory neurotransmitter of the brain. A neuron that releases GABA is called a gabaergic neuron. It plays a key role in the processes described in this book: without GABA, there would be no decision-making (see Chapters 4 and 5).

Globus pallidus. Gabaergic nucleus of the basal ganglia. It is functionally divided into an internal part (often abbreviated GPi) which is one of the main output structures of the basal ganglia and an external part (GPe) that is useless[1]...

Glutamate. Main excitatory neurotransmitter of the central nervous system. A neuron that releases glutamate is called a glutamatergic neuron.

Glycine. Neurotransmitter inhibitor of the spinal cord. A neuron that releases glycine is called a glycinergic neuron.

GPe. Acronym for the external globus pallidus (see globus pallidus).

GPi. Acronym for the internal globus pallidus (see globus pallidus).

Heuristic value. A theory has a heuristic value when it is easily understood by a larger number.

Heuristics. Behavioural economists and cognitive psychologists use the term heuristics in judgement to describe intuitive mental operations that bias our reasoning (see Chapters 1 and 18).

[1] This is a private joke; there is more and more evidence to show that it plays a key role in the dynamic properties of the basal ganglia. Moreover, evolution rarely conserves useless structures (see Chapter 21).

Hippocampus. Anatomical structure belonging to the telencephalon located in the inner part of the temporal cortical lobe. Its name comes from the analogy that exists between its form and the sea horse (*hippocampus* in Latin). This structure is closely related to the cingulate network and plays a key role in memory and mental representation (see Chapter 12).

Hyper-direct pathway. Pathway between the cortex and the GPi that passes through the NST. Its influence is excitatory: its activation increases the activity of GPi neurons (see Fig. 7.2).

Indirect pathway. Pathway between the cortex and the GPi that passes through the striatum, the GPe and the NST. Its influence is excitatory: its activation increases the activity of GPi neurons (see Fig. 7.2).

Interneuron. Neuron that connects with one (or more) other neuron(s) of the same structure. It is found in particular in the cortical structures and in the striatum.

k-armed bandits. Experimental paradigm for studying the learning and decision-making processes. They are so called in reference to the nicknames of the slot machines in the US. The one-armed bandit designates a protocol in which the subject must associate an action (press a lever for example) with a reward whose contingency rule is statistical (for example, rewarded on average once in three trials) and implicit (that is, it ignores its value at the origin). In the plural, it designates a protocol in which the subject has to choose between two (two-armed-bandit task, in English) or several (k-armed bandit task) actions whose contingency rules are different. The optimum behaviour is to test the different options first to estimate their respective expectations, then focus on the action associated with the highest expectation. Herrnstein showed that it was almost never the adopted behaviour (see Chapter 1).

Lottery. An experimental paradigm in which the subject has to choose between several options whose contingency rules are statistical (for example, rewarded once every three trials on average) and explicit (i.e. the subject knows the value). In economics, lotteries are used to study the behaviour of individuals faced with multiple choices. It can be 'real' lotteries (choose between A, where you have two chances out of three to win 100 €, and B, where you have one chance out of three to win 200 €); or, it can be more abstract lotteries (choose between a policy that sacrifices 200 people out of 600, or another where there is one chance out of three that the 600 will die). Fortunately (or unfortunately, it depends on the case), most of the time, subjects do not experience the consequences of their choices in this type of experiment!

Medium spiny neuron. Projection neuron of the striatum. There is a tendency to call them striatal projection neurons (SPN).

Mesencephalon. Deep subdivision of the brain that consists of the tectum, raphe nucleus, and tegmentum.

Motor loop. Subdivision of the telencephalic loop in charge of motor behaviour in mammals (see Fig. 17.2).

Myotome. Muscular segment of the lamprey body whose alternating contraction is responsible for its displacement.

Neurotransmitter. Molecule that transmits information between two neurons at their contact area called the synapse. The neurotransmitter is released into the extracellular space between the two neurons, called the synaptic cleft, by the pre-synaptic neuron and binds to receptors located on the postsynaptic neuron. This chemical message will be retransformed by this binding into an electric message. There are excitatory neurotransmitters: their fixation leads to an increase in the firing frequency of the postsynaptic neuron, and inhibitory neurotransmitters which have the opposite effect.

Oculomotor loop. Subdivision of the telencephalic loop which controls the gaze orientation in mammals (see Fig. 17.2).

Orbitofrontal loop. Subdivision of the telencephalic loop involved in cognition in mammals (see Figs. 17.2 and 19.1). The orbitofrontal network is rudimentary in rodents and develops mainly in primates.

Pallium. The anterior and dorsal mantle of the telencephalon in anamniotes, reptiles, and birds. It is organized into three layers.

Peripheral nervous system. Nerves and ganglia located outside the central nervous system whose function is to relay information between the former and the body.

Prefrontal network. Subdivision of the telencephalic loop involved in the advanced decision-making process in mammals (see Figs. 17.2 and 19.1). The prefrontal circuit is rudimentary in rodents and develops mainly in primates.

Projection neuron. Neuron of a structure (cortical area or sub-cortical nucleus) that connects with one (or more) neuron(s) of one (or more) other structure(s).

Pyramidal neuron projection. Neuron of cortical areas.

Scalar. Used here in the sense of numerical value.

SNc. Acronym for substantia nigra pars compacta.

SNr. Acronym for substantia nigra pars reticulata.

Spikes/s. Abbreviation for action potentials per second which is the unit of measurement for the firing rate of neurons. As a first approximation it can be considered that information transmitted to a neuron is coded by its firing rate (see Chapter 3).

Striatum. The largest nucleus of the basal ganglia. It consists in several populations of gabaergic and cholinergic neurons. It is the main entrance structure of the basal ganglia. Its complex architecture gives it rich properties, all of which are still not well understood, but as a simplification in our approach, we have reduced it to a single population of neurons. It is at the striatal level that reinforcement learning processes take place in vertebrates (see Chapter 5).

Subiculum. Subdivision of the hippocampus.

Substantia nigra. Nucleus of the mesencephalon that is functionally divided into two distinct structures. The substantia nigra pars reticulata is gabaergic and it is one of the output structures of the basal ganglia involved in the oculomotor loop. The substantia nigra pars compacta is mainly dopaminergic. It is the main source of dopamine released into the brain (see Chapter 6).

Subthalamic nucleus. The only nucleus of the basal ganglia, of which it forms one of the input structures, consisting of glutamatergic neurons.

Synaptic gain. The strength of the connection between two neurons is called synaptic gain: the greater the gain, the greater the influence of the pre-synaptic neuron on the postsynaptic neuron. Sometimes we also talk about synaptic coupling.

Telencephalic loop. Network formed by the cortex, the basal ganglia, and the thalamus. It is a neologism because there is no existing terminology to coin it. Its architecture is described in Figs. 8.2 and 17.2.

Telencephalon. Anterior subdivision of the brain. It consists of the olfactory bulb, pallidum striatum, and pallium (sometimes called mantle) which, in mammals, the dorsal and anterior part of is called the cortex and the ventral hippocampus. It was long believed that the development of the telencephalon was characteristic of mammals, but it is now known that it develops similarly in other taxon such as fishes and birds.

Thalamus. Subcortical nucleus which plays a key role as an interface between the sensory and the executive systems.

Utility function. Often shortened to utility (U). This is a logarithmic function that modulates the value given to an option based on its probability of occurrence. It has been formalized by Bernouilli and is used in economics to model the preferences of individuals (see Chapter 1).

Ventral tegmental area. Dopaminergic nucleus of the mesencephalon. It is functionally associated with the substantia nigra pars compacta. The ventral tegmental area innervates the prefrontal, orbitofrontal, and cingulate loops, whereas the substantia nigra pars compacta releases dopamine into the motor and oculomotor networks.

VTA. Acronym for ventral tegmental area.

Bibliography

Agid Y (1991) Parkinson's disease: pathophysiology. *Lancet* 337:1321–1323.

Albin RL, Young AB, Penney JB (1989) The functional anatomy of basal ganglia disorders. *Trends Neurosci* 12:366–375.

Albin RL, Young AB, Penney JB (1995) The functional anatomy of disorders of the basal ganglia. *Trends Neurosci* 18:63–64.

Albouy G, King BR, Maquet P, Doyon J (2013) Hippocampus and striatum: dynamics and interaction during acquisition and sleep-related motor sequence memory consolidation. *Hippocampus* 23:985–1004.

Alexander GE, Crutcher MD (1990) Functional architecture of basal ganglia circuits: neural substrates of parallel processing. *Trends Neurosci* 13:266–271.

Alexander ME, Wickens JR (1993) Analysis of striatal dynamics: the existence of two modes of behaviour. *J Theor Biol* 163:413–438.

Amemiya S, Noji T, Kubota N, Nishijima T, Kita I (2014) Noradrenergic modulation of vicarious trial-and-error behavior during a spatial decision-making task in rats. *Neuroscience* 265:291–301.

Andari E, Duhamel J-R, Zalla T, Herbrecht E, Leboyer M, Sirigu A (2010) Promoting social behavior with oxytocin in high-functioning autism spectrum disorders. *Proc Natl Acad Sci* 107:4389–4394.

Andersen P, Morris RG, Amaral D, Bliss T, O'Keefe J (2007) *The Hippocampus Book*. Oxford: Oxford University Press.

Anderson P, Lomo T (1966) Mode of activation of hippocampal pyramidal cells by excitatory synapses on dendrites. *Exp Brain Res* 2:247–260.

Annese J, Schenker-Ahmed NM, Bartsch H, Maechler P, Sheh C, Thomas N, Kayano J, Ghatan A, Bresler N, Frosch MP, Klaming R, Corkin S (2014) Postmortem examination of patient H.M.'s brain based on histological sectioning and digital 3D reconstruction. *Nat Commun* 5:3122.

Apicella P, Scarnati E, Ljungberg T, Schultz W (1992) Neuronal activity in monkey striatum related to the expectation of predictable environmental events. *J Neurophysiol* 68:945–960.

Apicella P, Ravel S, Sardo P, Legallet E (1998) Influence of predictive information on responses of tonically active neurons in the monkey striatum. *J Neurophysiol* 80:3341–3344.

Arbuthnott GW, Ingham CA, Wickens JR (2000) Dopamine and synaptic plasticity in the neostriatum. *J Anat* 196 (Pt 4):587–596.

Ariely D (2008) *Predictably Irrational: The Hidden Forces that Shape our Decisions*. New York: Harper.

Aubert I, Ghorayeb I, Normand E, Bloch B (2000) Phenotypical characterization of the neurons expressing the D1 and D2 dopamine receptors in the monkey striatum. *J Comp Neurol* 418:22–32.

Azouz R, Gray CM (1999) Cellular mechanisms contributing to response variability of cortical neurons in vivo. *J Neurosci* 19:2209–2223.

Baddeley AD (1993) La mémoire humaine théorie et pratique trad. de l'anglais sous la dir. de Solange Hollard. Grenoble: Presses universitaires de Grenoble.

Bagneux V, Bollon T, Dantzer C (2012) Do (un)certainty appraisal tendencies reverse the influence of emotions on risk taking in sequential tasks? *Cogn Emot* 26:568–576.

Bar-Gad I, Bergman H (2001) Stepping out of the box: information processing in the neural networks of the basal ganglia. *Curr Opin Neurobiol* 11:689–695.

Barbeau A (1972) Role of dopamine in the nervous system. *Monogr Hum Genet* 6:114–136.

Barron AB, Sovik E, Cornish JL (2010) The roles of dopamine and related compounds in reward-seeking behavior across animal phyla. *Front Behav Neurosci* 4:163.

Barry C, Burgess N (2014) Neural mechanisms of self-location. *Curr Biol* 24:R330–339.

Bechara A, Damasio H, Damasio AR (2000) Emotion, decision making and the orbitofrontal cortex. *Cereb Cortex* 10:295–307.

Bechara A, Damasio AR, Damasio H, Anderson SW (1994) Insensitivity to future consequences following damage to human prefrontal cortex. *Cognition* 50:7–15.

Bechara A, Tranel D, Damasio H, Damasio AR (1996) Failure to respond autonomically to anticipated future outcomes following damage to prefrontal cortex. *Cereb Cortex* 6:215–225.

Bedecarrats A, Cornet C, Simmers J, Nargeot R (2013) Implication of dopaminergic modulation in operant reward learning and the induction of compulsive-like feeding behavior in Aplysia. *Learn Mem* 20:318–327.

Bekoff M, Byers JA (1998) *Animal Play: Evolutionary, Comparative, and Ecological Perspectives*. Cambridge, UK: Cambridge University Press.

Berkowitz BA (1983) Dopamine and dopamine receptors as target sites for cardiovascular drug action. *Fed Proc* 42:3019–3021.

Bernardi G (2012) The use of tools by wrasses (Labridae). *Coral Reefs* 31:39–39.

Bernoulli D (1738) Specimen theoriae novae de mensura sortis. In: *Commentarii Academiae scientiarum imperialis Petropolitanae*. V. 1738, pp. 175–192. St-Petersburg.

Bertran-Gonzalez J, Herve D, Girault JA, Valjent E (2010) What is the degree of segregation between striatonigral and striatopallidal projections? *Front Neuroanat* 4:136–145.

Blumenthal A, Steiner A, Seeland K, Redish AD (2011) Effects of pharmacological manipulations of NMDA-receptors on deliberation in the Multiple-T task. *Neurobiol Learn Mem* 95:376–384.

Boraud T, Bezard E, Bioulac B, Gross CE (2001) Action selection in parkinsonian akinesia. In: 7th Triennial Meeting of the International-Basal-Ganglia-Society (Nicholson LFB, Faull RLM, eds), pp 13–18. Waitangi, New Zealand.

Boraud T, Bezard E, Bioulac B, Gross CE (2002) From single extracellular unit recording in experimental and human parkinsonism to the development of a functional concept of the role played by the basal ganglia in motor control. *Prog Neurobiol* 66:205–283.

Boraud T, Brown P, Goldberg JA, Graybiel AM, Magill PJ (2005) Oscillations in the basal ganglia: the good, the bad, and the unexpected. In: *Basal Ganglia VIII* (Bolam JP, Ingham CA, Magill PJ, eds), pp 3–24. New York: Springer.

Boraud T, Leblois A, Rougier NP (2018) A natural history of skills. *Prog Neurobiol* 71:114–124.Bouton ME (2007) *Learning and Behavior: A Contemporary Synthesis*. Sunderland, MA: Sinaur Associates.

Bradshaw CM, Szabadi E, Bevan P, Ruddle HV (1979) The effect of signaled reinforcement availability on concurrent performances in humans. *J Exp Anal Behav* 32:65–74.

Brass M, Furstenberg A, Mele AR (2019) Why neuroscience does not disprove free will. *Neurosci Biobehav Rev* 102:251–263.

Broglie LD (1956) *Nouvelles perspectives en microphysique*. Paris: Albin Michel.

Brown P (2003) Oscillatory nature of human basal ganglia activity: relationship to the pathophysiology of Parkinson's disease. *Mov Disord* 18:357–363.

Bueti D, Walsh V, Frith C, Rees G (2008) Different brain circuits underlie motor and perceptual representations of temporal intervals. *J Cogn Neurosci* 20:204–214.

Buhusi CV, Meck WH (2005) What makes us tick? Functional and neural mechanisms of interval timing. *Nat Rev Neurosci* 6:755–765.

Burbaud P et al. (2013) Neuronal activity correlated with checking behaviour in the subthalamic nucleus of patients with obsessive-compulsive disorder. *Brain* 136:304–317.

Bures J, Fenton AA, Kaminsky Y, Zinyuk L (1997) Place cells and place navigation. *Proc Natl Acad Sci U S A* 94:343–350.

Buser P, Debru C (2011) *Le temps, instant et durée de la philosophie aux neurosciences*. Paris: O. Jacob.

Bustos G, Abarca J, Campusano J, Bustos V, Noriega V, Aliaga E (2004) Functional interactions between somatodendritic dopamine release, glutamate receptors and brain-derived neurotrophic factor expression in mesencephalic structures of the brain. *Brain Res Rev* 47:126–144.

Cachope R, Cheer JF (2014) Local control of striatal dopamine release. *Front Behav Neurosci* 8:188.

Caggiano V, Fogassi L, Rizzolatti G, Thier P, Casile A (2009) Mirror neurons differentially encode the peripersonal and extrapersonal space of monkeys. *Science* 324:403–406.

Calabresi P, Picconi B, Tozzi A, Di Filippo M (2007) Dopamine-mediated regulation of corticostriatal synaptic plasticity. *Trends Neurosci* 30:211–219.

Call J, Tomasello M (2008) Does the chimpanzee have a theory of mind? 30 years later. *Trends Cogn Sci* 12:187–192.

Calvin WH, Stevens CF (1968) Synaptic noise and other sources of randomness in motoneuron interspike intervals. *J Neurophysiol* 31:574–587.

Canfield JG, Mizumori SJ (2004) Methods for chronic neural recording in the telencephalon of freely behaving fish. *J Neurosci Methods* 133:127–134.

Caplin A, Dean M (2008) Axiomatic methods, dopamine and reward prediction error. *Curr Opin Neurobiol* 18:197–202.

Caporale N, Dan Y (2008) Spike timing-dependent plasticity: a Hebbian learning rule. *Annu Rev Neurosci* 31:25–46.

Cavanna AE, Servo S, Monaco F, Robertson MM (2009) The behavioral spectrum of Gilles de la Tourette syndrome. *J Neuropsychiatry Clin Neurosci* 21:13–23.

Centonze D, Gubellini P, Pisani A, Bernardi G, Calabresi P (2003a) Dopamine, acetylcholine and nitric oxide systems interact to induce corticostriatal synaptic plasticity. *Rev Neurosci* 14:207–216.

Centonze D, Grande C, Saulle E, Martin AB, Gubellini P, Pavon N, Pisani A, Bernardi G, Moratalla R, Calabresi P (2003b) Distinct roles of D1 and D5 dopamine receptors in motor activity and striatal synaptic plasticity. *J Neurosci* 23:8506–8512.

Chang L, Fang Q, Zhang S, Poo M-m, Gong N (2015) Mirror-induced self-directed behaviors in rhesus monkeys after visual-somatosensory training. *Curr Biol* 25:212–217.

Cisek P (2006) Integrated neural processes for defining potential actions and deciding between them: a computational model. *J Neurosci* 26:9761-9770.

Cnotka J, Gunturkun O, Rehkamper G, Gray RD, Hunt GR (2008) Extraordinary large brains in tool-using New Caledonian crows (*Corvus moneduloides*). *Neurosci Lett* 433:241–245.

Cohen NJ, Eichenbaum H, Deacedo BS, Corkin S (1985) Different memory systems underlying acquisition of procedural and declarative knowledge. *Ann N Y Acad Sci* 444:54–71.

Coles P (1988) Benveniste controversy rages on in the French press. *Nature* 334:372.

Coles P (1989) Benveniste controversy. INSERM closes the file. *Nature* 340:178.

Contreras D, Timofeev I, Steriade M (1996) Mechanisms of long-lasting hyperpolarizations underlying slow sleep oscillations in cat corticothalamic networks. *J Physiol* 494 (Pt 1):251–264.

Coricelli G, Nagel R (2009) Neural correlates of depth of strategic reasoning in medial prefrontal cortex. *Proc Natl Acad Sci U S A* 106:9163–9168.

Coricelli G, Critchley HD, Joffily M, O'Doherty JP, Sirigu A, Dolan RJ (2005) Regret and its avoidance: a neuroimaging study of choice behavior. *Nat Neurosci* 8:1255–1262.

Corkin S (2002) What's new with the amnesic patient H.M.? *Nat Rev Neurosci* 3:153–160.

Cottrell GA (1967) Occurrence of dopamine and noradrenaline in the nervous tissue of some invertebrate species. *Br J Pharmacol Chemother* 29:63–69.

Cowan N (1988) Evolving conceptions of memory storage, selective attention, and their mutual constraints within the human information-processing system. *Psychol Bull* 104:163–191.

Creese I, Sibley DR, Leff S, Hamblin M (1981) Dopamine receptors: subtypes, localization and regulation. *Fed Proc* 40:147–152.

Crosby G (2015) *Fight, Flight, Freeze : Taming Your Reptilian Brain and Other Practical Approaches to Self-Improvement*. Seattle, USA: Crosbyod Publishing.

Dallerac GM, Vatsavayai SC, Cummings DM, Milnerwood AJ, Peddie CJ, Evans KA, Walters SW, Rezaie P, Hirst MC, Murphy KP (2011) Impaired long-term potentiation in the prefrontal cortex of Huntington's disease mouse models: rescue by D1 dopamine receptor activation. *Neurodegener Dis* 8:230–239.

Daw ND (2007) Dopamine: at the intersection of reward and action. *Nat Neurosci* 10:1505–1507.

Daw ND, Niv Y, Dayan P (2005) Uncertainty-based competition between prefrontal and dorsolateral striatal systems for behavioral control. *Nat Neurosci* 8:1704–1711.

Daw ND, O'Doherty JP, Dayan P, Seymour B, Dolan RJ (2006) Cortical substrates for exploratory decisions in humans. *Nature* 441:876–879.

Dayan P, Niv Y, Seymour B, Daw ND (2006) The misbehavior of value and the discipline of the will. *Neural Netw* 19:1153–1160.

de Veer MW, Gallup GG, Jr., Theall LA, van den Bos R, Povinelli DJ (2003) An 8-year longitudinal study of mirror self-recognition in chimpanzees (Pan troglodytes). *Neuropsychologia* 41:229–234.

de Waal F (2006) *Le Singe en nous*. Paris: Fayard.

Deco G, Rolls ET, Romo R (2009) Stochastic dynamics as a principle of brain function. *Prog Neurobiol* 88:1–16.

Degos B, Deniau JM, Chavez M, Maurice N (2009) Chronic but not acute dopaminergic transmission interruption promotes a progressive increase in cortical beta frequency synchronization: relationships to vigilance state and akinesia. *Cereb Cortex* 19:1616–1630.

Dejean C, Gross CE, Bioulac B, Boraud T (2008) Dynamic changes in the cortex-basal ganglia network after dopamine depletion in the rat. *J Neurophysiol* 100:385–396.

Dejean C, Nadjar A, Le Moine C, Bioulac B, Gross CE, Boraud T (2012) Evolution of the dynamic properties of the cortex-basal ganglia network after dopaminergic depletion in rats. *Neurobiol Dis* 46:402–413.

Del Arco A, Mora F (2009) Neurotransmitters and prefrontal cortex-limbic system interactions: implications for plasticity and psychiatric disorders. *J Neural Transm* 116:941–952.

Delfour F, Marten K (2001) Mirror image processing in three marine mammal species: killer whales (*Orcinus orca*), false killer whales (*Pseudorca crassidens*) and California sea lions (*Zalophus californianus*). *Behav Processes* 53:181–190.

Delgado MR, Li J, Schiller D, Phelps EA (2008) The role of the striatum in aversive learning and aversive prediction errors. *Philos Trans R Soc Lond B Biol Sci* 363:3787–3800.

DeLong MR (1990) Primate models of movement disorders of basal ganglia origin. *Trends Neurosci* 13:281–285.

Deng W, Aimone JB, Gage FH (2010) New neurons and new memories: how does adult hippocampal neurogenesis affect learning and memory? *Nat Rev Neurosci* 11:339–350.

Deng YP, Lei WL, Reiner A (2006) Differential perikaryal localization in rats of D1 and D2 dopamine receptors on striatal projection neuron types identified by retrograde labeling. *J Chem Neuroanat* 32:101–116.

Deniau JM, Chevalier G (1984) Synaptic organization of the basal ganglia: an electroanatomical approach in the rat. *Ciba Found Symp* 107:48–63.

Deniau JM, Chevalier G (1985) Disinhibition as a basic process in the expression of striatal functions. II The striato-nigral influence on thalamo-cortical cells of the ventromedial thalamic nucleus. *Brain Res* 335:227–233.

Dennett DC (1991) *Consciousness Explained*. Boston: Little Brown.

Descartes R (1658) *Discours de la methode pour bien conduire sa raison, et chercher la verité dans les sciences, plus la dioptrique et les météores*. Paris: H. Le Gras.

Diamond J (1997) *Guns, Germs and Steel the Fates of Human Societies*. New York: Norton.

Ding L, Perkel DJ (2004) Long-term potentiation in an avian basal ganglia nucleus essential for vocal learning. *J Neurosci* 24:488–494.

Dougan JD, McSweeney FK, Farmer VA (1985) Some parameters of behavioral contrast and allocation of interim behavior in rats. *J Exp Anal Behav* 44:325–335.

Doya K (2000) Reinforcement learning in continuous time and space. *Neural Comput* 12:219–245.

Dubuc R, Brocard F, Antri M, Fenelon K, Gariepy JF, Smetana R, Menard A, Le Ray D, Viana Di Prisco G, Pearlstein E, Sirota MG, Derjean D, St-Pierre M, Zielinski B, Auclair F, Veilleux D (2008) Initiation of locomotion in lampreys. *Brain Res Rev* 57:172–182.

Eagle DM, Bari A, Robbins TW (2008) The neuropsychopharmacology of action inhibition: cross-species translation of the stop-signal and go/no-go tasks. *Psychopharmacology* 199:439–456.

Ekstrom AD, Kahana MJ, Caplan JB, Fields TA, Isham EA, Newman EL, Fried I (2003) Cellular networks underlying human spatial navigation. *Nature* 425:184–188.

Emery NJ (2006) Cognitive ornithology: the evolution of avian intelligence. *Philos Trans R Soc Lond B Biol Sci* 361:23–43.

Ericsson J, Silberberg G, Robertson B, Wikstrom MA, Grillner S (2011) Striatal cellular properties conserved from lampreys to mammals. *J Physiol* 589:2979–2992.

Ericsson J, Stephenson-Jones M, Perez-Fernandez J, Robertson B, Silberberg G, Grillner S (2013) Dopamine differentially modulates the excitability of striatal neurons of the direct and indirect pathways in lamprey. *J Neurosci* 33:8045–8054.

Fabbri-Destro M, Rizzolatti G (2008) Mirror neurons and mirror systems in monkeys and humans. *Physiology* (Bethesda) 23:171–179.

Feldman DE (2012) The spike-timing dependence of plasticity. *Neuron* 75:556–571.

Fernando AB, Murray JE, Milton AL (2013) The amygdala: securing pleasure and avoiding pain. *Front Behav Neurosci* 7:190.

Feyerabend P (1979) *Contre la méthode esquisse d'une théorie anarchiste de la connaissance traduit de l'anglais par Baudouin Jurdant et Agnès Schlumberger*. Paris: Éditions du Seuil.

Fink GR, Halligan PW, Marshall JC, Frith CD, Frackowiak RS, Dolan RJ (1996) Where in the brain does visual attention select the forest and the trees? *Nature* 382:626–628.

Fino E, Venance L (2011) Spike-timing dependent plasticity in striatal interneurons. *Neuropharmacology* 60:780–788.

Fiorillo CD, Tobler PN, Schultz W (2003) Discrete coding of reward probability and uncertainty by dopamine neurons. *Science* 299:1898–1902.

Fitoussi A, Dellu-Hagedorn F, De Deurwaerdere P (2013) Monoamines tissue content analysis reveals restricted and site-specific correlations in brain regions involved in cognition. *J Neurosci* 255:233–245.

Flaubert G (2008) *Dictionnaire des idées reçues*. Paris: Librio.

Florian RV (2007) Reinforcement learning through modulation of spike-timing-dependent synaptic plasticity. *Neural Comput* 19:1468–1502.

Fouquet C, Tobin C, Rondi-Reig L (2010) A new approach for modeling episodic memory from rodents to humans: the temporal order memory. *Behav Brain Res* 215:172–179.

Frank MJ, Samanta J, Moustafa AA, Sherman SJ (2007) Hold your horses: impulsivity, deep brain stimulation, and medication in parkinsonism. *Science* 318:1309–1312.

Freed DM, Corkin S (1988) Rate of forgetting in H.M.: 6-month recognition. *Behav Neurosci* 102:823–827.

Freed DM, Corkin S, Cohen NJ (1987) Forgetting in H.M.: a second look. *Neuropsychologia* 25:461–471.

Frohman LA (1983) CNS peptides and glucoregulation. *Annu Rev Physiol* 45:95–107.

Fuxe K, Borroto-Escuela DO, Romero-Fernandez W, Zhang WB, Agnati LF (2013) Volume transmission and its different forms in the central nervous system. *Chin J Integr Med* 19:323–329.

Gage GJ, Stoetzner CR, Wiltschko AB, Berke JD (2010) Selective activation of striatal fast-spiking interneurons during choice execution. *Neuron* 67:466–479.

Gale SD, Perkel DJ (2010) Anatomy of a songbird basal ganglia circuit essential for vocal learning and plasticity. *J Chem Neuroanat* 39:124–131.

Gallagher M, McMahan RW, Schoenbaum G (1999) Orbitofrontal cortex and representation of incentive value in associative learning. *J Neurosci* 19:6610–6614.

Gallese V, Fadiga L, Fogassi L, Rizzolatti G (1996) Action recognition in the premotor cortex. *Brain* 119 (Pt 2):593–609.

Ganos C, Roessner V, Münchau A (2013) The functional anatomy of Gilles de la Tourette syndrome. *Neurosci Biobehav Rev* 37:1050–1062.

Garenne A, Pasquereau B, Guthrie M, Bioulac B, Boraud T (2011) Basal Ganglia preferentially encode context dependent choice in a two-armed bandit task. *Front Syst Neurosci* 5:23.

Georgopoulos AP et al. (1982) On the relations between the direction of two-dimensional arm movements and cell discharge in primate motor cortex. *J Neurosci* 2(11):1527–37.

Gerfen CR, Keefe KA (1994) Neostriatal dopamine receptors. *Trends Neurosci* 17:2–3; author reply 4–5.

Gerfen CR, Engber TM, Mahan LC, Susel Z, Chase TN, Monsma FJ, Jr., Sibley DR (1990) D1 and D2 dopamine receptor-regulated gene expression of striatonigral and striatopallidal neurons. *Science* 250:1429–1432.

Ghanbarian E, Motamedi F (2013) Ventral tegmental area inactivation suppresses the expression of CA1 long term potentiation in anesthetized rat. *PLoS One* 8:e58844.

Gilbert-Norton LB, Shahan TA, Shivik JA (2009) Coyotes (*Canis latrans*) and the matching law. *Behav Processes* 82:178–183.

Goldberg LI, Volkman PH, Kohli JD (1978) A comparison of the vascular dopamine receptor with other dopamine receptors. *Annu Rev Pharmacol Toxicol* 18:57–79.

Goss AE, Wischner GJ (1956) Vicarious trial and error and related behavior. *Psychol Bull* 53:35–54.

Graft DA, Lea SE, Whitworth TL (1977) The matching law in and within groups of rats. *J Exp Anal Behav* 27:183–194.

Granado N, Ortiz O, Suarez LM, Martin ED, Cena V, Solis JM, Moratalla R (2008) D1 but not D5 dopamine receptors are critical for LTP, spatial learning, and LTP-Induced arc and zif268 expression in the hippocampus. *Cereb Cortex* 18:1–12.

Graybiel AM, Aosaki T, Flaherty AW, Kimura M (1994) The basal ganglia and adaptive motor control. *Science* 265:1826–1831.

Groves PM (1983) A theory of the functional organization of the neostriatum and the neostriatal control of voluntary movement. *Brain Res* 286:109–132.

Guehl D, Benazzouz A, Aouizerate B, Cuny E, Rotge JY, Rougier A, Tignol J, Bioulac B, Burbaud P (2008) Neuronal correlates of obsessions in the caudate nucleus. *Biol Psychiatry* 63:557–562.

Gupta DS (2014) Processing of sub- and supra-second intervals in the primate brain results from the calibration of neuronal oscillators via sensory, motor and feedback processes. *Frontiers in Psychology* 5.

Guthrie M, Leblois A, Garenne A, Boraud T (2013) Interaction between cognitive and motor cortico-basal ganglia loops during decision making: a computational study. *J Neurophysiol* 109:3025–3040.

Haber SN, Fudge JL, McFarland NR (2000) Striatonigrostriatal pathways in primates form an ascending spiral from the shell to the dorsolateral striatum. *J Neurosci* 20:2369–2382.Haber SN, Knutson B (2010) The reward circuit: linking primate anatomy and human imaging. *Neuropsychopharmacol* 35:4–26.

Hansel D, Sompolinsky H (1992) Synchronization and computation in a chaotic neural network. *Phys Rev Lett* 68:718–721.

Hansel D, Sompolinsky H (1993) Solvable model of spatiotemporal chaos. *Phys Rev Lett* 71:2710–2713.

Hanson VD (1990) *Le Modèle occidental de la guerre la bataille d'infanterie dans la Grèce classique préf. de John Keegan trad. par Alain Billault*. Paris: Les Belles lettres.

Hanson VD (2002) *Carnage et culture les grandes batailles qui ont fait l'Occident trad. de l'anglais par Pierre-Emmanuel Dauzat*. Paris: Flammarion.

Hardman CD, Henderson JM, Finkelstein DI, Horne MK, Paxinos G, Halliday GM (2002) Comparison of the basal ganglia in rats, marmosets, macaques, baboons, and humans: volume and neuronal number for the output, internal relay, and striatal modulating nuclei. *J Comp Neurol* 445:238–255.

Harmer SL, Panda S, Kay SA (2001) Molecular bases of circadian rhythms. *Annu Rev Cell Dev Biol* 17:215–253.

Harrington DL, Haaland KY, Hermanowicz N (1998a) Temporal processing in the basal ganglia. *Neuropsychology* 12:3–12.

Harrington DL, Haaland KY, Knight RT (1998b) Cortical networks underlying mechanisms of time perception. *J Neurosci* 18:1085–1095.

Hebb DO (1949) *The Organization of Behavior: A Neuropsychological Theory*. New York: Wiley.

Heitz PU (1979) The neuroendocrine system of the gastrointestinal tract. *Pathol Res Pract* 165:333–348.

Herculano-Houzel S (2009) The human brain in numbers: a linearly scaled-up primate brain. *Front Hum Neurosci* 3:31.

Herculano-Houzel S (2011a) Not all brains are made the same: new views on brain scaling in evolution. *Brain Behav Evol* 78:22–36.

Herculano-Houzel S (2011b) Brains matter, bodies maybe not: the case for examining neuron numbers irrespective of body size. *Ann N Y Acad Sci* 1225:191–199.

Herculano-Houzel S (2012a) Neuronal scaling rules for primate brains: the primate advantage. *Prog Brain Res* 195:325–340.

Herculano-Houzel S (2012b) The remarkable, yet not extraordinary, human brain as a scaled-up primate brain and its associated cost. *Proc Natl Acad Sci U S A* 109 Suppl 1:10661–10668.

Herculano-Houzel S (2014) The glia/neuron ratio: how it varies uniformly across brain structures and species and what that means for brain physiology and evolution. *Glia* 62:1377–1391.

Herculano-Houzel S, Mota B, Lent R (2006) Cellular scaling rules for rodent brains. *Proc Natl Acad Sci U S A* 103:12138–12143.

Herculano-Houzel S, Collins CE, Wong P, Kaas JH (2007) Cellular scaling rules for primate brains. *Proc Natl Acad Sci U S A* 104:3562–3567.Herculano-Houzel S, Ribeiro P, Campos L, Valotta da Silva A, Torres LB, Catania KC, Kaas JH (2011) Updated neuronal scaling rules for the brains of Glires (rodents/lagomorphs). *Brain Behav Evol* 78:302–314.Herculano-Houzel S, Watson C, Paxinos G (2013) Distribution of neurons in functional areas of the mouse cerebral cortex reveals quantitatively different cortical zones. *Front Neuroanat* 7:35.

Herrnstein RJ (1974) Formal properties of the matching law. *J Exp Anal Behav* 21:159–164.

Herrnstein RJ, Vaughan W, Jr., Mumford DB, Kosslyn SM (1989) Teaching pigeons an abstract relational rule: insideness. *Percept Psychophys* 46:56–64.

Hirano T, Best P, Olds J (1970) Units during habituation, discrimination learning, and extinction. *Electroencephalogr Clin Neurophysiol* 28:127–135.

Hobbes T (1999) *Les questions concernant la liberté, la nécéssité et le hasard: controverse avec Bramhall, II*. Paris: J. Vrin.

Hong S, Hikosaka O (2011) Dopamine-mediated learning and switching in cortico-striatal circuit explain behavioral changes in reinforcement learning. *Front Behav Neurosci* 5:15.

Hori E, Nishio Y, Kazui K, Umeno K, Tabuchi E, Sasaki K, Endo S, Ono T, Nishijo H (2005) Place-related neural responses in the monkey hippocampal formation in a virtual space. *Hippocampus* 15:991–996.

Hornykiewicz O (1966) Dopamine and brain function. *Pharmacol Rev* 18:925–964.

Hornykiewicz O (1974) The mechanism of action of L-dopa in Parkinson's disease. *Life Sci* 15:1249–1259.

Horvitz JC (2000) Mesolimbocortical and nigrostriatal dopamine responses to salient non-reward events. *Neuroscience* 96:651–656.

Houk JC, Adams JL, Gurney K (1995) A model of how the basal ganglia generate and use neural signals that predict reinforcement. In: *Models of Information Processing in the Basal Ganglia* (Houk JC, Davis JL, Beiser DG, eds). Cambridge, MA: MIT press.

Houthakker HS (1950) Revealed preference and the utility function. *Economics* 17:159–174.

Howard R (2001) Un homme d'exception.

Hu D, Amsel A (1995) A simple test of the vicarious trial-and-error hypothesis of hippocampal function. *Proc Natl Acad Sci U S A* 92:5506–5509.

Huang YY, Levine A, Kandel DB, Yin D, Colnaghi L, Drisaldi B, Kandel ER (2014) D1/D5 receptors and histone deacetylation mediate the Gateway Effect of LTP in hippocampal dentate gyrus. *Learn Mem* 21:153–160.

Humphries MD, Khamassi M, Gurney K (2012) Dopaminergic control of the exploration-exploitation trade-off via the basal ganglia. *Front Neurosci* 6:9.

Iordanova MD (2009) Dopaminergic modulation of appetitive and aversive predictive learning. *Rev Neurosci* 20:383–404.

Jaeger D, Gilman S, Alridge JW (1995) Neuronal activity in the striatum and pallidum of primates related to the execution of externally cued reaching movements. *Brain Res* 694:111–127.

Jarrell TA, Wang Y, Bloniarz AE, Brittin CA, Xu M, Thomson JN, Albertson DG, Hall DH, Emmons SW (2012) The connectome of a decision-making neural network. *Science* 337:437–444.

Jovanic T, Schneider-Mizell CM, Shao M, Masson J-B, Denisov G, Fetter RD, Mensh BD, Truman JW, Cardona A, Zlatic M (2016) Competitive disinhibition mediates behavioral choice and sequences in Drosophila. *Cell* 167:858–870.

Kable JW, Glimcher PW (2009) The neurobiology of decision: consensus and controversy. *Neuron* 63:733–745.

Kahneman D (2012) *Système 1, système 2 les deux vitesses de la pensée traduit de l'anglais (États-Unis) par Raymond Clarinard*. Paris: Flammarion.

Kahneman D, Tversky A (1979) Prospect Theory: an analysis of decision under risk. *Econometrica* 47:263–291.

Kanno T (1977) Physiology of paraneurons. *Arch Histol Jpn* 40 Suppl:13–29.

Keegan J (1996) *Histoire de la guerre du néolithique à la guerre du Golfe*. Paris: Ed. Dagorno.

Kerr JN, Wickens JR (2001) Dopamine D-1/D-5 receptor activation is required for long-term potentiation in the rat neostriatum in vitro. *J Neurophysiol* 85:117–124.

Khamassi M, Humphries MD (2012) Integrating cortico-limbic-basal ganglia architectures for learning model-based and model-free navigation strategies. *Front Behav Neurosci* 6:79.

Killeen PR (2011) Models of trace decay, eligibility for reinforcement, and delay of reinforcement gradients, from exponential to hyperboloid. *Behav Processes* 87:57–63.

Kimura M, Kato M, Shimazaki H, Watanabe K, Matsumoto N (1996) Neural information transferred from the putamen to the globus pallidus during learned movement in the monkey. *J Neurophysiol* 76:3771–3786.

Kindt KS, Quast KB, Giles AC, De S, Hendrey D, Nicastro I, Rankin CH, Schafer WR (2007) Dopamine mediates context-dependent modulation of sensory plasticity in C. elegans. *Neuron* 55:662–676.

Kircher TT, Senior C, Phillips ML, Rabe-Hesketh S, Benson PJ, Bullmore ET, Brammer M, Simmons A, Bartels M, David AS (2001) Recognizing one's own face. *Cognition* 78:B1–B15.

Kobayashi S, Pinto de Carvalho O, Schultz W (2010) Adaptation of reward sensitivity in orbitofrontal neurons. *J Neurosci* 30:534–544.

Kohn AF (1997) Computer simulation of noise resulting from random synaptic activities. *Comput Biol Med* 27:293–308.

Koike N, Yoo S-H, Huang H-C, Kumar V, Lee C, Kim T-K, Takahashi JS (2012) Transcriptional architecture and chromatin landscape of the core circadian clock in mammals. *Science* 338:349–354.

Koos T, Tepper JM, Wilson CJ (2004) Comparison of IPSCs evoked by spiny and fast-spiking neurons in the neostriatum. *J Neurosci* 24:7916–7922.

Kotter R, Wickens J (1995) Interactions of glutamate and dopamine in a computational model of the striatum. *J Comput Neurosci* 2:195–214.

Krawczyk M, Mason X, De Backer J, Sharma R, Normandeau CP, Hawken ER, Di Prospero C, Chiang C, Martinez A, Jones AA, Doudnikoff E, Caille S, Bezard E, Georges F, Dumont EC (2013) D1 dopamine receptor-mediated LTP at GABA synapses encodes motivation to self-administer cocaine in rats. *J Neurosci* 33:11960–11971.

Lampl I, Reichova I, Ferster D (1999) Synchronous membrane potential fluctuations in neurons of the cat visual cortex. *Neuron* 22:361–374.

Laquitaine S, Piron C, Abellanas D, Loewenstein Y, Boraud T (2013) Complex population response of dorsal putamen neurons predicts the ability to learn. *PLoS One* 8:e80683.

Larsson LI (1980a) Gastrointestinal cells producing endocrine, neurocrine and paracrine messengers. *Clin Gastroenterol* 9:485–516.

Larsson LI (1980b) On the possible existence of multiple endocrine, paracrine and neurocrine messengers in secretory cell systems. *Invest Cell Pathol* 3:73–85.

Lau B, Glimcher PW (2005) Dynamic response-by-response models of matching behavior in rhesus monkeys. *J Exp Anal Behav* 84:555–579.

Lau B, Glimcher PW (2008) Value representations in the primate striatum during matching behavior. *Neuron* 58:451–463.

Le Moine C, Bloch B (1995) D1 and D2 dopamine receptor gene expression in the rat striatum: sensitive cRNA probes demonstrate prominent segregation of D1 and D2 mRNAs in distinct neuronal populations of the dorsal and ventral striatum. *J Comp Neurol* 355:418–426.

Leblois A (2006) Rôle de la compétition entre boucles fermées dans la dynamique du réseau extrapyramidal: approches neurophysique et neurophysiologique. Available at: http://www.theses.fr/2006PA066194

Leblois A, Boraud T, Meissner W, Bergman H, Hansel D (2006) Competition between feedback loops underlies normal and pathological dynamics in the basal ganglia. *J Neurosci* 26:3567–3583.

Leblois A, Perkel DJ (2012) Striatal dopamine modulates song spectral but not temporal features through D1 receptors. *Eur J Neurosci* 35:1771–1781.

Lemon N, Manahan-Vaughan D (2006) Dopamine D1/D5 receptors gate the acquisition of novel information through hippocampal long-term potentiation and long-term depression. *J Neurosci* 26:7723–7729.

Lerner JS, Keltner D (2001) Fear, anger, and risk. *J Pers Soc Psychol* 81:146–159.

Lerner JS, Li Y, Weber EU (2013) The financial costs of sadness. *Psychol Sci* 24:72–79.

Lerner JS, Li Y, Valdesolo P, Kassam K (2014) Emotion and Decision Making. *Annu Rev Psychol*.

Lesburgueres E, Bontempi B (2011) Mecanismes de consolidation de la memoire: importance de l'etiquetage precoce des neurones du neocortex. *Med Sci* (Paris) 27:1048–1050.

Lesburgueres E, Gobbo OL, Alaux-Cantin S, Hambucken A, Trifilieff P, Bontempi B (2011) Early tagging of cortical networks is required for the formation of enduring associative memory. *Science* 331:924–928.

Lethmate J, Ducker G (1973) Studies on self-recognition in a mirror in orangutans, chimpanzees, gibbons and various other monkey species. *Z Tierpsychol* 33:248–269.

Libet B (1999) Do we have free will? *J Conscious Stud* 6:47–57.

Logan CJ, Jelbert SA, Breen AJ, Gray RD, Taylor AH (2014) Modifications to the Aesop's fable paradigm change New Caledonian crow performances. *PLoS One* 9:e103049.

Mackintosh NJ (1974) *The Psychology of Animal Learning*. London and New York: Academic Press.

MacLean PD (1973) *An Evolutionary Approach to the Investigation of Psychoneuro-Endocrine Functions*. New York: Plenum Press.

Marc-Aurèle (1995) *Pensées pour moi-même trad. du grec par Frédérique Vervliet Suivi de Sur Marc-Aurèle*. Paris: Arléa diff. le Seuil.

Matsuzawa T, Tomogana M, Tanaka M (2006) *Cognitive Development in Chimpanzees*. Japan: Springer Verlag.

Matthews LR, Temple W (1979) Concurrent schedule assessment of food preference in cows. *J Exp Anal Behav* 32:245–254.

McClellan AD, Grillner S (1984) Activation of 'fictive swimming' by electrical microstimulation of brainstem locomotor regions in an in vitro preparation of the lamprey central nervous system. *Brain Res* 300:357–361.

McDonald RJ, Hong NS (2013) How does a specific learning and memory system in the mammalian brain gain control of behavior? *Hippocampus* 23:1084–1102.

Menard A, Grillner S (2008) Diencephalic locomotor region in the lamprey--afferents and efferent control. *J Neurophysiol* 100:1343–1353.

Miller JF, Neufang M, Solway A, Brandt A, Trippel M, Mader I, Hefft S, Merkow M, Polyn SM, Jacobs J, Kahana MJ, Schulze-Bonhage A (2013) Neural activity in human hippocampal formation reveals the spatial context of retrieved memories. *Science* 342:1111–1114.

Milner B (1959) The memory defect in bilateral hippocampal lesions. *Psychiatr Res Rep Am Psychiatr Assoc* 11:43–58.

Milner B (1972) Disorders of learning and memory after temporal lobe lesions in man. *Clin Neurosurg* 19:421–446.

Milner B, Penfield W (1955) The effect of hippocampal lesions on recent memory. *Trans Am Neurol Assoc*:42–48.

Monsma FJ, Jr., McVittie LD, Gerfen CR, Mahan LC, Sibley DR (1989) Multiple D2 dopamine receptors produced by alternative RNA splicing. *Nature* 342:926–929.

Mooney R (1995) Behavioral learning: the illuminated songbird. *Curr Biol* 5:609–611.

Morris G, Arkadir D, Nevet A, Vaadia E, Bergman H (2004) Coincident but distinct messages of midbrain dopamine and striatal tonically active neurons. *Neuron* 43:133–143.

Morris G, Nevet A, Arkadir D, Vaadia E, Bergman H (2006) Midbrain dopamine neurons encode decisions for future action. *Nat Neurosci* 9:1057–1063.

Morris RG, Garrud P, Rawlins JN, O'Keefe J (1982) Place navigation impaired in rats with hippocampal lesions. *Nature* 297:681–683.

Muenzinger KF (1956) On the origin and early use of the term vicarious trial and error (VTE). *Psychol Bull* 53:493–494.

Muller RU, Stead M, Pach J (1996) The hippocampus as a cognitive graph. *J Gen Physiol* 107:663–694.

Nagel R (1995) Unraveling in guessing games: an experimental study. *American Economic Review* 85:1313–1326.

Nambu A, Tokuno H, Hamada I, Kita H, Imanishi M, Akazawa T, Ikeuchi Y, Hasegawa N (2000) Excitatory cortical inputs to pallidal neurons via the subthalamic nucleus in the monkey. *J Neurophysiol* 84:289–300.

Nambu A, Tokuno H, Takada M (2002) Functional significance of the cortico-subthalamo-pallidal 'hyperdirect' pathway. *Neurosci Res* 43:111–117.

Nargeot R, Baxter DA, Patterson GW, Byrne JH (1999) Dopaminergic synapses mediate neuronal changes in an analogue of operant conditioning. *J Neurophysiol* 81:1983–1987.

Nargeot R, Simmers J (2011) Neural mechanisms of operant conditioning and learning-induced behavioral plasticity in Aplysia. *Cell Mol Life Sci* 68:803–816.

Nevet A, Morris G, Saban G, Arkadir D, Bergman H (2007) Lack of spike-count and spike-time correlations in the substantia nigra reticulata despite overlap of neural responses. *J Neurophysiol* 98:2232–2243.

Newsome WT, Britten KH, Movshon JA (1989) Neuronal correlates of a perceptual decision. *Nature* 341:52–54.

Nielsen JA, Zielinski BA, Ferguson MA, Lainhart JE, Anderson JS (2013) An evaluation of the left-brain vs. right-brain hypothesis with resting state functional connectivity magnetic resonance imaging. *PLoS ONE* 8:e71275.

Nisbett RE, Zukier H, Lemley RE (1981) The dilution effect: nondiagnostic information weakens the implications of diagnostic information. *Cog Psych* 13:248–277.

Nisenbaum ES, Wilson CJ (1995) Potassium currents responsible for inward and outward rectification in rat neostriatal spiny projection neurons. *J Neurosci* 15:4449–4463.

Nogues X, Corsini MM, Marighetto A, Abrous DN (2012) Functions for adult neurogenesis in memory: an introduction to the neurocomputational approach and to its contribution. *Behav Brain Res* 227:418–425.

Norman KA (2010) How hippocampus and cortex contribute to recognition memory: revisiting the complementary learning systems model. *Hippocampus* 20:1217–1227.

Nottebohm F, Alvarez-Buylla A, Cynx J, Kirn J, Ling CY, Nottebohm M, Suter R, Tolles A, Williams H (1990) Song learning in birds: the relation between perception and production. *Philos Trans R Soc Lond B Biol Sci* 329:115–124.

Nowak LG, Sanchez-Vives MV, McCormick DA (1997) Influence of low and high frequency inputs on spike timing in visual cortical neurons. *Cereb Cortex* 7:487–501.

Nunes EJ, Randall PA, Podurgiel S, Correa M, Salamone JD (2013) Nucleus accumbens neurotransmission and effort-related choice behavior in food motivation: effects of drugs acting on dopamine, adenosine, and muscarinic acetylcholine receptors. *Neurosci Biobehav Rev* 37:2015–2025.

O'Kane G, Kensinger EA, Corkin S (2004) Evidence for semantic learning in profound amnesia: an investigation with patient H.M. *Hippocampus* 14:417–425.

O'Keefe J, Dostrovsky J (1971) The hippocampus as a spatial map: preliminary evidence from unit activity in the freely-moving rat. *Brain Res* 34:171–175.

Obeso JA, Rodriguez-Oroz MC, Stamelou M, Bhatia KP, Burn DJ (2014) The expanding universe of disorders of the basal ganglia. *Lancet* 384:523–531.

Obeso JA, Jahanshahi M, Alvarez L, Macias R, Pedroso I, Wilkinson L, Pavon N, Day B, Pinto S, Rodriguez-Oroz MC, Tejeiro J, Artieda J, Talelli P, Swayne O, Rodriguez R, Bhatia K, Rodriguez-Diaz M, Lopez G, Guridi J, Rothwell JC (2009) What can man do without basal ganglia motor output? The effect of combined unilateral subthalamotomy and pallidotomy in a patient with Parkinson's disease. *Exp Neurol* 220:283–292.

Oorschot DE (1996) Total number of neurons in the neostriatal, pallidal, subthalamic, and substantia nigral nuclei of the rat basal ganglia: a stereological study using the cavalieri and optical disector methods. *J Comp Neurol* 366:580–599.

Pakkenberg B, Gundersen HJ (1997) Neocortical neuron number in humans: effect of sex and age. *J Comp Neurol* 384:312–320.

Pakkenberg B, Pelvig D, Marner L, Bundgaard MJ, Gundersen HJ, Nyengaard JR, Regeur L (2003) Aging and the human neocortex. *Exp Gerontol* 38:95–99.

Palminteri S, Boraud T, Lafargue G, Dubois B, Pessiglione M (2009) Brain hemispheres selectively track the expected value of contralateral options. *J Neurosci* 29:13465–13472.

Papale AE, Stott JJ, Powell NJ, Regier PS, Redish AD (2012) Interactions between deliberation and delay-discounting in rats. *Cogn Affect Behav Neurosci* 12:513–526.

Papousek H, Papousek M (1974) Mirror image and self-recognition in young human infants: I. A method of experimental analysis. *Dev Psychobiol* 7:149–157.

Pare D, Shink E, Gaudreau H, Destexhe A, Lang EJ (1998) Impact of spontaneous synaptic activity on the resting properties of cat neocortical pyramidal neurons In vivo. *J Neurophysiol* 79:1450–1460.

Parent A, Hazrati L-N (1993) Anatomical aspects of information processing in primate basal ganglia. *Trends Neurosci* 16:111–116.

Parent A, Hazrati L-N (1995a) Functional anatomy of the basal ganglia. II. The place of subthalamic nucleus and external pallidum in basal ganglia circuitry. *Brain Res Rev* 20:128–154.

Parent A, Hazrati L-N (1995b) Functional anatomy of the basal ganglia. I. The cortico-basal ganglia-thalamo-cortical loop. *Brain Res Rev* 20:91–127.

Parent A, Hazrati L-N, Smith Y (1989) The subthalamic nucleus in primates. A neuroanatomical and immunohistochemical study. *Curr Probl Neurol* 9:29–35.

Parent A, Cote PY, Lavoie B (1995) Chemical anatomy of primate basal ganglia. *Prog Neurobiol* 46:131–197.

Parent A, Sato F, Wu Y, Gauthier J, Levesque M, Parent M (2000) Organization of the basal ganglia: the importance of axonal collateralization. *Trends Neurosci* 23:S20–27.

Parkinson J (1817) *An Essay on the Shaking Palsy*. London: Sherwood, Nelly and Jones.

Pascal B (1936) *Oeuvres Complètes*. Paris, France: Gallimard.

Pasquereau B, Nadjar A, Arkadir D, Bezard E, Goillandeau M, Bioulac B, Gross CE, Boraud T (2007) Shaping of motor responses by incentive values through the basal ganglia. *J Neurosci* 27:1176–1183.

Pawlak V, Kerr JN (2008) Dopamine receptor activation is required for corticostriatal spike-timing-dependent plasticity. *J Neurosci* 28:2435–2446.

Paz R, Boraud T, Natan C, Vaadia E, Bergman H (2003) Learning induced visuomotor competition in the primary motor cortex. *Nat Neurosci* 6:882–890.

Penfield W, Milner B (1958) Memory deficit produced by bilateral lesions in the hippocampal zone. *AMA Arch Neurol Psychiatry* 79:475–497.

Perez-Fernandez J, Stephenson-Jones M, Suryanarayana SM, Robertson B, Grillner S (2014) Evolutionarily conserved organization of the dopaminergic system in lamprey: SNc/VTA afferent and efferent connectivity and D2 receptor expression. *J Comp Neurol* 522:3775–3794.

Pessiglione M, Seymour B, Flandin G, Dolan RJ, Frith CD (2006) Dopamine-dependent prediction errors underpin reward-seeking behaviour in humans. *Nature* 442:1042–1045.

Pessiglione M, Petrovic P, Daunizeau J, Palminteri S, Dolan RJ, Frith CD (2008) Subliminal instrumental conditioning demonstrated in the human brain. *Neuron* 59:561–567.

Piron C, Kase D, Topalidou M, Goillandeau M, Orignac H, N'Guyen TH, Rougier N, Boraud T (2016) The globus pallidus pars interna in goal-oriented and routine behaviors: resolving a long-standing paradox. *Mov Disord* 31:1146–1154.

Plotnik JM, de Waal FB, Reiss D (2006) Self-recognition in an Asian elephant. *Proc Natl Acad Sci U S A* 103:17053–17057.

Postel J (1966) The mirror test in the study of the relationships of the aged person with his image. *Bull Inst Natl Sante Rech Med* 21:611–623.

Povinelli DJ, Rulf AB, Landau KR, Bierschwale DT (1993) Self-recognition in chimpanzees (Pan troglodytes): distribution, ontogeny, and patterns of emergence. *J Comp Psychol* 107:347–372.

Prather JF, Peters S, Nowicki S, Mooney R (2008) Precise auditory-vocal mirroring in neurons for learned vocal communication. *Nature* 451:305–310.

Preston SD, de Waal FB (2002) Empathy: its ultimate and proximate bases. *Behav Brain Sci* 25:1–20; discussion 20–71.

Prior H, Schwarz A, Gunturkun O (2008) Mirror-induced behavior in the magpie (Pica pica): evidence of self-recognition. *PLoS Biol* 6:e202.

Ranck JB, Jr. (1973) Studies on single neurons in dorsal hippocampal formation and septum in unrestrained rats: I. Behavioral correlates and firing repertoires. *Exp Neurol* 41:461–531.

Rao SM, Harrington DL, Haaland KY, Bobholz JA, Cox RW, Binder JR (1997) Distributed neural systems underlying the timing of movements. *J Neurosci* 17:5528–5535.

Rascol O (2000) Medical treatment of levodopa-induced dyskinesias. *Ann Neurol* 47:S179–188.

Reichelt AC, Lee JL (2013) Memory reconsolidation in aversive and appetitive settings. *Front Behav Neurosci* 7:118.

Reiner A, Medina L, Veenman CL (1998) Structural and functional evolution of the basal ganglia in vertebrates. *Brain Res Rev* 28:235–285.

Rescorla RA, Wagner AR (1972) A theory of Pavlovian conditioning: variations in the effectiveness of reinforcement and nonreinforcement. In: *Classical Conditioning II* (Black AH, Prokasy WF, eds), pp 64–99. Appleton-Century-Crofts. New York, NY, USA.

Retailleau A, Boraud T (2014) The Michelin red guide of the brain: role of dopamine in goal-oriented navigation. *Front Syst Neurosci* 8:32.

Retailleau A, Morris G (2018) Spatial rule learning and corresponding CA1 place cell reorientation depend on local dopamine release. *Curr Biol* 28:ahead of print.

Retailleau A, Bardy A-S, Thomas B (submitted) Newts can learn but are not humdrum.

Retailleau A, Etienne S, Guthrie M, Boraud T (2012) Where is my reward and how do I get it? Interaction between the hippocampus and the basal ganglia during spatial learning. *J Physiol Paris* 106:72–80.

Retailleau A, Dejean C, Fourneaux B, Leinekugel X, Boraud T (2013) Why am I lost without dopamine? Effects of 6-OHDA lesion on the encoding of reward and decision process in CA3. *Neurobiol Dis* 59:151–164.

Rice ME, Cragg SJ (2008) Dopamine spillover after quantal release: rethinking dopamine transmission in the nigrostriatal pathway. *Brain Res Rev* 58:303–313.

Rich EL, Wallis JD (2013) Prefrontal-amygdala interactions underlying value coding. *Neuron* 80:1344–1346.

Rizzolatti G, Fadiga L, Gallese V, Fogassi L (1996) Premotor cortex and the recognition of motor actions. *Cogn Brain Res* 3:131–141.

Rizzolatti G, Fadiga L, Fogassi L, Gallese V (1999) Resonance behaviors and mirror neurons. *Arch Ital Biol* 137:85–100.

Robertson GS, Jian M (1995) D1 and D2 dopamine receptors differentially increase Fos-like immunoreactivity in accumbal projections to the ventral pallidum and midbrain. *Neuroscience* 64:1019–1034.

Robertson MM (2011) Gilles de la Tourette syndrome: the complexities of phenotype and treatment. *Br J Hosp Med (Lond)* 72:100–107.

Rodriguez F, Lopez JC, Vargas JP, Broglio C, Gomez Y, Salas C (2002) Spatial memory and hippocampal pallium through vertebrate evolution: insights from reptiles and teleost fish. *Brain Res Bull* 57:499–503.

Rogerson T, Cai DJ, Frank A, Sano Y, Shobe J, Lopez-Aranda MF, Silva AJ (2014) Synaptic tagging during memory allocation. *Nat Rev Neurosci* 15:157–169.

Roggenhofer E, Fidzinski P, Shor O, Behr J (2013) Reduced threshold for induction of LTP by activation of dopamine D1/D5 receptors at hippocampal CA1-subiculum synapses. *PLoS One* 8:e62520.

Roggenhofer E, Fidzinski P, Bartsch J, Kurz F, Shor O, Behr J (2010) Activation of dopamine D1/D5 receptors facilitates the induction of presynaptic long-term potentiation at hippocampal output synapses. *Eur J Neurosci* 32:598–605.

Rolls ET (2010) A computational theory of episodic memory formation in the hippocampus. *Behav Brain Res* 215:180–196.

Rotge JY, Langbour N, Jaafari N, Guehl D, Bioulac B, Aouizerate B, Allard M, Burbaud P (2010) Anatomical alterations and symptom-related functional activity in obsessive-compulsive disorder are correlated in the lateral orbitofrontal cortex. *Biol Psychiatry* 67:e37–38.

Rotge JY, Aouizerate B, Amestoy V, Lambrecq V, Langbour N, Nguyen TH, Dovero S, Cardoit L, Tignol J, Bioulac B, Burbaud P, Guehl D (2012) The associative and limbic thalamus in the pathophysiology of obsessive-compulsive disorder: an experimental study in the monkey. *Transl Psychiatry* 2:e161.

Rubin A, Yartsev MM, Ulanovsky N (2014) Encoding of head direction by hippocampal place cells in bats. *J Neurosci* 34:1067–1080.

Rudebeck PH, Mitz AR, Chacko RV, Murray EA (2013) Effects of amygdala lesions on reward-value coding in orbital and medial prefrontal cortex. *Neuron* 80:1519–1531.

Rutledge RB, Dean M, Caplin A, Glimcher PW (2011) Testing the reward prediction error hypothesis with an axiomatic model. *J Neurosci* 30:13525–13536.

Ryczko D, Gratsch S, Auclair F, Dube C, Bergeron S, Alpert MH, Cone JJ, Roitman MF, Alford S, Dubuc R (2013) Forebrain dopamine neurons project down to a brainstem region controlling locomotion. *Proc Natl Acad Sci U S A* 110:E3235–3242.

Sage JR, Anagnostaras SG, Mitchell S, Bronstein JM, De Salles A, Masterman D, Knowlton BJ (2003) Analysis of probabilistic classification learning in patients with Parkinson's disease before and after pallidotomy surgery. *Learn Mem* 10:226–236.

Saito H, Katahira K, Okanoya K, Okada M (2011) Statistical mechanics of structural and temporal credit assignment effects on learning in neural networks. *Phys Rev E Stat Nonlin Soft Matter Phys* 83:051125.

Salamone JD, Correa M (2012) The mysterious motivational functions of mesolimbic dopamine. *Neuron* 76:470–485.

Samejima K, Doya K (2007) Multiple representations of belief states and action values in corticobasal ganglia loops. *Ann N Y Acad Sci* 1104:213–228.

Samejima K, Ueda Y, Doya K, Kimura M (2005) Representation of action-specific reward values in the striatum. *Science* 310:1337–1340.

Samuelson PA (1938) A note on the pure theory of consumer behavior. *Economia* 1:61–71.

Sandstrom MI, Rebec GV (2003) Characterization of striatal activity in conscious rats: contribution of NMDA and AMPA/kainate receptors to both spontaneous and glutamate-driven firing. *Synapse* 47:91–100.

Schmidt B, Papale A, Redish AD, Markus EJ (2013) Conflict between place and response navigation strategies: effects on vicarious trial and error (VTE) behaviors. *Learn Mem* 20:130–138.

Schmolck H, Kensinger EA, Corkin S, Squire LR (2002) Semantic knowledge in patient H.M. and other patients with bilateral medial and lateral temporal lobe lesions. *Hippocampus* 12:520–533.

Schotanus SM, Chergui K (2008) Dopamine D1 receptors and group I metabotropic glutamate receptors contribute to the induction of long-term potentiation in the nucleus accumbens. *Neuropharmacology* 54:837–844.

Schultz W (1998a) Predictive reward signal of dopamine neurons. *J Neurophysiol*:1–27.

Schultz W (1998b) Predictive reward signal of dopamine neurons. *J Neurophysiol* 80:1–27.

Schultz W (2006) Behavioral theories and the neurophysiology of reward. *Annu Rev Psychol* 57:87–115.

Schultz W, Dayan P, Montague PR (1997) A neural substrate of prediction and reward. *Science* 275:1593–1599.

Scoville WB, Milner B (1957) Loss of recent memory after bilateral hippocampal lesions. *J Neurol Neurosurg Psychiatry* 20:11–21.

Sesack SR, Hawrylak VA, Melchitzky DS, Lewis DA (1998) Dopamine innervation of a subclass of local circuit neurons in monkey prefrontal cortex: ultrastructural analysis of tyrosine hydroxylase and parvalbumin immunoreactive structures. *Cereb Cortex* 8:614–622.

Sescousse G, Redoute J, Dreher JC (2010) The architecture of reward value coding in the human orbitofrontal cortex. *J Neurosci* 30:13095–13104.

Sescousse G, Li Y, Dreher JC (2014) A common currency for the computation of motivational values in the human striatum. *Soc Cogn Affect Neurosci* 10:467–473.

Sescousse G, Barbalat G, Domenech P, Dreher JC (2013) Imbalance in the sensitivity to different types of rewards in pathological gambling. *Brain* 136:2527–2538.

Seth AK, Izhikevich E, Reeke GN, Edelman GM (2006) Theories and measures of consciousness: an extended framework. *Proc Natl Acad Sci U S A* 103:10799–10804.

Seymour B, Dolan R (2008) Emotion, decision making, and the amygdala. *Neuron* 58:662–671.

Shadlen Michael N, Kiani R (2013) Decision making as a window on cognition. *Neuron* 80:791–806.

Shakespeare W (1606 [2006]) *MacBeth*. Paris: Flammarion.

Shannon CE (1948) A mathematical theory of communication. *The Bell System Technical Journal* 27:623–656.

Sharot T (2011) *The Optimism Bias: A Tour of the Irrationally Positive Brain*. New York: Pantheon Books.

Shepherd GM (2011) The microcircuit concept applied to cortical evolution: from three-layer to six-layer cortex. *Front Neuroanat* 5:30.

Shibasaki M, Ishida M (2012) Effects of overtraining on extinction in newts (*Cynops pyrrhogaster*). *J Comp Psychol* 126:368–371.

Sibley DR, Monsma FJ, Jr., McVittie LD, Gerfen CR, Burch RM, Mahan LC (1992) Molecular neurobiology of dopamine receptor subtypes. *Neurochem Int* 20 Suppl:17s–22s.

Simon H (1947) *Administrative Behavior*. New York: Macmillan.

Simon HA (1955) A behavioral model of rational choice. *The Quarterly Journal of Economics* 69:99–118.

Sloman SA (1996) The empirical case for two systems of reasoning. *Psychol Bull* 119:3–22.

Smith A (1778) *Recherches sur la nature et les causes de la richesse des nations traduit de l'anglais de M. Adam Smith*. La Haye.

Snider SR, Kuchel O (1983) Dopamine: an important neurohormone of the sympathoadrenal system. Significance of increased peripheral dopamine release for the human stress response and hypertension. *Endocr Rev* 4:291–309.

Soon CS, He AH, Bode S, Haynes JD (2013) Predicting free choices for abstract intentions. *Proc Natl Acad Sci U S A* 110:6217–6222.

Spinoza BD (2000) *Ethics*. Oxford and New York: Oxford University Press.

Squire LR (2004) Memory systems of the brain: a brief history and current perspective. *Neurobiol Learn Mem* 82:171–177.

Squire LR, Kandel ER (2009) *Memory: From Mind to Molecules*, 2nd Edition. Greenwood Village: Roberts & Co.

Steiner AP, Redish AD (2012) The road not taken: neural correlates of decision making in orbitofrontal cortex. *Front Neurosci* 6:131.

Stephenson-Jones M, Ericsson J, Robertson B, Grillner S (2012) Evolution of the basal ganglia: dual-output pathways conserved throughout vertebrate phylogeny. *J Comp Neurol* 520:2957–2973.

Stephenson-Jones M, Kardamakis AA, Robertson B, Grillner S (2013) Independent circuits in the basal ganglia for the evaluation and selection of actions. *Proc Natl Acad Sci U S A* 110:E3670–3679.

Striedter GE (2017) *The Evolution of the Nervous System in Nonmammalian Vertebrates*, 2nd Edition. Amsterdam and Boston: Academic Press.

Suarez LM, Bustamante J, Orensanz LM, Martin del Rio R, Solis JM (2014) Cooperation of taurine uptake and dopamine D1 receptor activation facilitates the induction of protein synthesis-dependent late LTP. *Neuropharmacology* 79:101–111.

Sugiura M, Watanabe J, Maeda Y, Matsue Y, Fukuda H, Kawashima R (2005) Cortical mechanisms of visual self-recognition. *Neuroimage* 24:143–149.

Suri RE, Bargas J, Arbib MA (2001) Modeling functions of striatal dopamine modulation in learning and planning. *Neuroscience* 103:65–85.

Surmeier DJ, Eberwine J, Wilson CJ, Cao Y, Stefani A, Kitai ST (1992) Dopamine receptor subtypes colocalize in rat striatonigral neurons. *Proc Natl Acad Sci U S A* 89:10178–10182.

Sutton RS, Barto AG (1998) *Reinforcement Learning: An Introduction*. Cambridge, MA: MIT Press.

Svenningsson P, Fredholm BB, Bloch B, Le Moine C (2000) Co-stimulation of D(1)/D(5) and D(2) dopamine receptors leads to an increase in c-fos messenger RNA in cholinergic interneurons and a redistribution of c-fos messenger RNA in striatal projection neurons. *Neuroscience* 98:749–757.

Swanson LW (1995) Mapping the human brain: past, present, and future. *Trends Neurosci* 18:471–474.

Syed EC, Benazzouz A, Taillade M, Baufreton J, Champeaux K, Falgairolle M, Bioulac B, Gross CE, Boraud T (2012) Oscillatory entrainment of subthalamic nucleus neurons and behavioural consequences in rodents and primates. *Eur J Neurosci* 36:3246–3257.

Taylor JG, Reichlin B (1951) Vicarious trial and error. *Psychol Rev* 58:389–402.

Tchernichovski O, Marcus G (2014) Vocal learning beyond imitation: mechanisms of adaptive vocal development in songbirds and human infants. *Curr Opin Neurobiol* 28c:42–47.

Thaler RH, Johnson EJ (1990) Gambling with the house money and trying to break even: the effect of prior outcomes on risky choice. *Management Science* 36:643–660.

The MC5 (1969) In: Kick out the Jams.

Thibault D, Loustalot F, Fortin GM, Bourque MJ, Trudeau LE (2013) Evaluation of D1 and D2 dopamine receptor segregation in the developing striatum using BAC transgenic mice. *PLoS One* 8:e67219.

Thobois S, Ardouin C, Schmitt E, Lhommee E, Klinger H, Xie J, Lagrange C, Kistner A, Aya Kombo M, Fleury V, Poisson A, Fraix V, Broussolle E, Pollak P, Krack P (2010) Behavioral disorders in Parkinson's disease: from pathophysiology to the mastery of dopaminergic treatment. *Rev Neurol* (Paris) 166:816–821.

Thomas Y (2007) The history of the memory of water. *Homeopathy* 96:151–157.

Tolman EC (1948) Cognitive maps in rats and men. *Psychol Rev* 55:189–208.

Tomasello M (2004) *Aux origines de la cognition humaine*. Paris: éditions Retz.

Topalidou M, Kase D, Boraud T, Rougier NP (2018) Dual Competition between the Basal Ganglia and the Cortex. eNeuro pii, 5: NEURO.0339-17.2018. https://www.eneuro.org/content/eneuro/5/6/ENEURO.0339-17.2018.full.pdf.

Tronson NC, Corcoran KA, Jovasevic V, Radulovic J (2012) Fear conditioning and extinction: emotional states encoded by distinct signaling pathways. *Trends Neurosci* 35:145–155.

Tulving E (1995) Organisation of memory: quo vadis? In: *The Cognitive Neurosciences* (Gazzaniga MS, ed). Cambridge, MA: MIT Press.

Uddin LQ, Kaplan JT, Molnar-Szakacs I, Zaidel E, Iacoboni M (2005) Self-face recognition activates a frontoparietal 'mirror' network in the right hemisphere: an event-related fMRI study. *Neuroimage* 25:926–935.

Van Essen DC, Dierker DL (2007) Surface-based and probabilistic atlases of primate cerebral cortex. *Neuron* 56:209–225.

Van Loon GR (1983) Plasma dopamine: regulation and significance. *Fed Proc* 42:3012–3018.

van Rooyen JM, Offermeier J (1981) Peripheral dopaminergic receptors. Physiological and pharmaceutical aspects of therapeutic importance. *S Afr Med J* 59:329–332.

Vassena E, Krebs RM, Silvetti M, Fias W, Verguts T (2014) Dissociating contributions of ACC and vmPFC in reward prediction, outcome, and choice. *Neuropsychologia* 59:112–123.

Vassiliades V, Cleanthous A, Christodoulou C (2011) Multiagent reinforcement learning: spiking and nonspiking agents in the iterated Prisoner's Dilemma. *IEEE Trans Neural Netw* 22:639–653.

Vincent J-D (1986) *La Biologie des passions*: Paris: O. Jacob.

Vinogradova OS, Semyonova TP, Konovalov VF (1970) Trace phenomena in the activity of hippocampus and mammilary body neurons. In: *Biology of Memory* (Pribram KH, Broadbent DE, eds). San Diego, CA: Academic Press.

Voltaire (1828) General Correspondence, fifth volume. London, UK: Ode and Wodon.

von Neumann J, Morgenstern O (1944) *Theory of Games and Economic Behavior.* Princeton, NJ: Princeton University Press.

Wallon H (1934) *Les Origines du caractère chez l'enfant, les préludes du sentiment de personnalité*. Paris: Boivin.

Wan X, Nakatani H, Ueno K, Asamizuya T, Cheng K, Tanaka K (2011) The neural basis of intuitive best next-move generation in board game experts. *Science* 331:341–346.

Wang HH, Li LY, Wang LW, Liang CC (2007) Morphological and histological studies on the telencephalon of the salamander *Onychodactylus fischeri*. *Neurosci Bull* 23:170–174.

Welter ML, Burbaud P, Fernandez-Vidal S, Bardinet E, Coste J, Piallat B, Borg M, Besnard S, Sauleau P, Devaux B, Pidoux B, Chaynes P, Tezenas du Montcel S, Bastian A, Langbour N, Teillant A, Haynes W, Yelnik J, Karachi C, Mallet L (2011) Basal ganglia dysfunction in OCD: subthalamic neuronal activity correlates with symptoms severity and predicts high-frequency stimulation efficacy. *Transl Psychiatry* 1:e5.

Wickens JR, Kotter R, Alexander ME (1995) Effects of local connectivity on striatal function: stimulation and analysis of a model. *Synapse* 20:281–298.

Wiescholleck V, Manahan-Vaughan D (2014) Antagonism of D1/D5 receptors prevents long-term depression (LTD) and learning-facilitated LTD at the perforant path-dentate gyrus synapse in freely behaving animals. *Hippocampus* 24:1615–1622.

Willemet R (2013) Reconsidering the evolution of brain, cognition, and behavior in birds and mammals. *Front Psychol* 4:396.

Wilson CJ, Groves PM (1981) Spontaneous firing patterns of identified spiny neurons in the rat neostriatum. *Brain Res* 220:67–80.

Woller A, Gonze D (2013) The bird circadian clock: insights from a computational model. *J Biol Rhythms* 28:390–402.

Wunderlich K, Dayan P, Dolan RJ (2012) Mapping value based planning and extensively trained choice in the human brain. *Nat Neurosci* 15:786–791.

Xu TX, Yao WD (2010) D1 and D2 dopamine receptors in separate circuits cooperate to drive associative long-term potentiation in the prefrontal cortex. *Proc Natl Acad Sci U S A* 107:16366–16371.

Yartsev MM, Ulanovsky N (2013) Representation of three-dimensional space in the hippocampus of flying bats. *Science* 340:367–372.

Zago L, Petit L, Mellet E, Jobard G, Crivello F, Joliot M, Mazoyer B, Tzourio-Mazoyer N (2016) The association between hemispheric specialization for language production and for spatial attention depends on left-hand preference strength. *Neuropsychologia* 93:394–406.

Zink CF, Pagnoni G, Martin-Skurski ME, Chappelow JC, Berns GS (2004) Human striatal responses to monetary reward depend on saliency. *Neuron* 42:509–517.

Zoli M, Torri C, Ferrari R, Jansson A, Zini I, Fuxe K, Agnati LF (1998) The emergence of the volume transmission concept. *Brain Res Rev* 26:136–147.

Zweifel LS, Argilli E, Bonci A, Palmiter RD (2008) Role of NMDA receptors in dopamine neurons for plasticity and addictive behaviors. *Neuron* 59:486–496.

Index

Figures are indicated by *f* following the page number

For the benefit of digital users, indexed terms that span two pages (e.g., 52–53) may, on occasion, appear on only one of those pages.

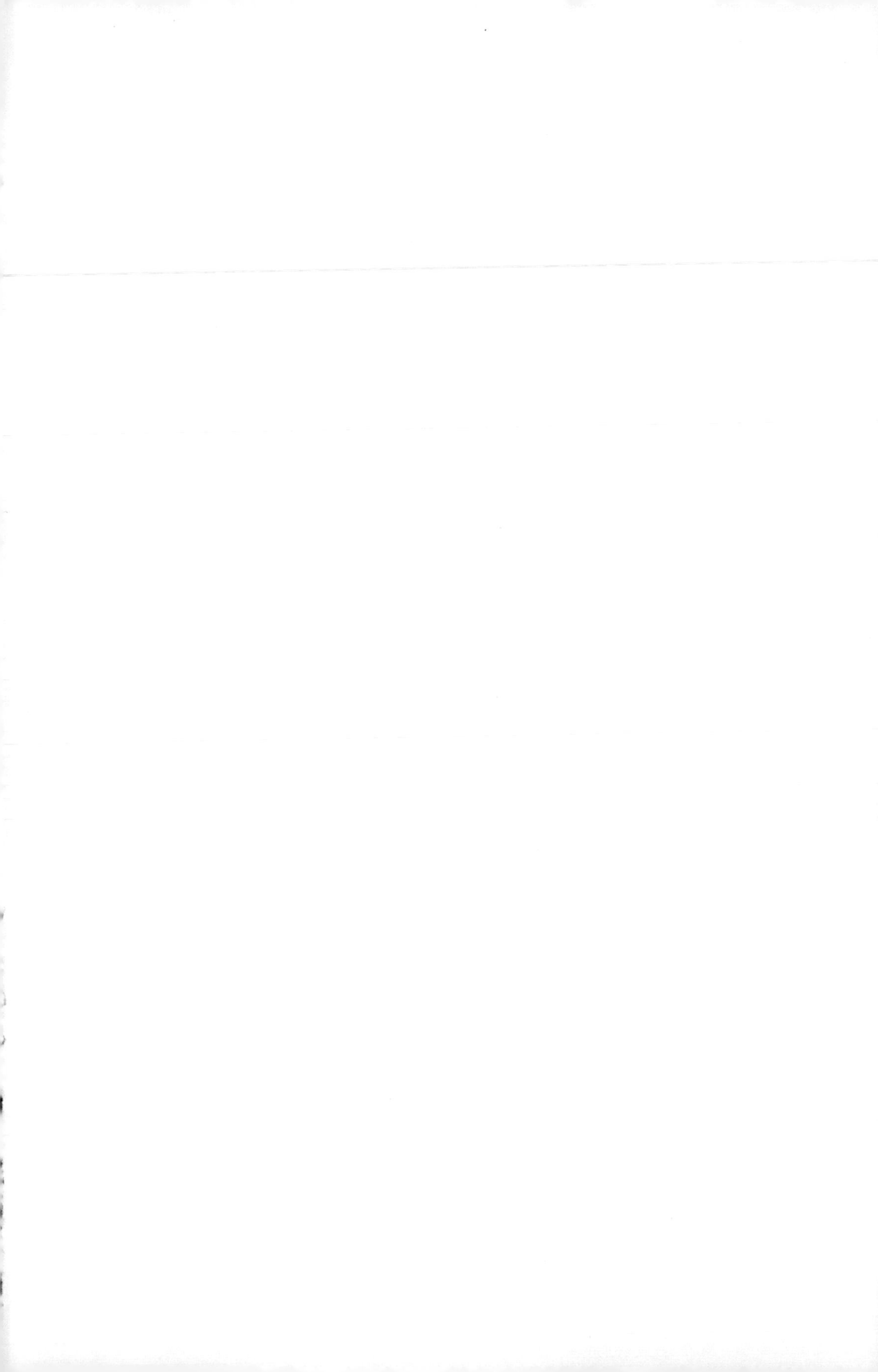